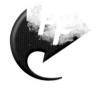

Fast Facts:
Smoking Cessation

Third edition

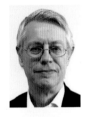

Robert West PhD
Professor of Health Psychology
Director of Tobacco Studies
Cancer Research UK Health Behaviour Research Centre
University College London
London, UK

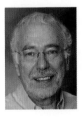

Saul Shiffman PhD
Research Professor of Clinical and
Health Psychology, Psychiatry, and
Pharmaceutical Sciences
University of Pittsburgh and Pinney Associates
Pittsburgh, Pennsylvania, USA

Declaration of Independence
This book is as balanced and as practical as we can make it.
Ideas for improvement are always welcome: feedback@fastfacts.com

HEALTH PRESS

Fast Facts: Smoking Cessation
First published 2004; second edition 2007
Third edition April 2016

Text © 2016 Robert West, Saul Shiffman
© 2016 in this edition Health Press Limited
Health Press Limited, Elizabeth House, Queen Street, Abingdon,
Oxford OX14 3LN, UK
Tel: +44 (0)1235 523233

Book orders can be placed by telephone or via the website. For regional distributors
or to order via the website, please go to: fastfacts.com

For telephone orders, please call +44 (0)1752 202301 (UK, Europe and Asia–
Pacific), 1 800 247 6553 (USA, toll free) or +1 419 281 1802 (Americas).

Fast Facts is a trademark of Health Press Limited.

The publisher and the authors have made every effort to ensure the accuracy of this
book, but cannot accept responsibility for any errors or omissions.

For all drugs, please consult the product labeling approved in your country for
prescribing information.

Registered names, trademarks, etc. used in this book, even when not marked as
such, are not to be considered unprotected by law.

A CIP record for this title is available from the British Library.

ISBN 978-1-908541-84-0

West R (Robert)
Fast Facts: Smoking Cessation/
Robert West, Saul Shiffman

Medical illustrations by Dee McLean, London.
Typesetting and page layout by Zed, Oxford, UK.
Printed by Hobbs the Printer Ltd, Totton, UK.

Glossary

Acetylcholine (ACh): a neurotransmitter; nicotine resembles ACh sufficiently to act at nicotinic ACh receptors located throughout the central and peripheral nervous systems

Addiction: often used synonymously with 'dependence' to mean a condition in which someone has impaired control over a reward-seeking activity. A slightly modified definition is preferred, in which 'addiction' is a chronic condition in which an unhealthy priority is attached to an activity because of a disordered motivational system, resulting in a repeated powerful motivation to engage in a maladaptive behavior

$\alpha_4\beta_2$ nicotinic acetylcholine receptor: the most common type of receptor in the brain to which nicotine binds, believed to be important in many of the addictive properties of nicotine

Behavioral support: a structured program of counseling and behavioral techniques aimed at helping smokers to stop smoking

Bupropion: a medication licensed as an aid to smoking cessation (brand names Zyban and Wellbutrin)

Cotinine: a metabolite of nicotine with a half-life in blood of 14–20 hours, which makes it a useful measure of the amount of nicotine taken in over the past few days

Counseling: in this context, targeted advice and support focused on maintaining or enhancing motivation to achieve and sustain abstinence, and on strategies for avoiding or coping with urges to smoke and withdrawal symptoms

Craving: experience of powerful motivation (urge, desire or need) to engage in a behavior

Cytisine: an alkaloid found in high concentrations in the plant *Cytisus laburnum*. It acts as a partial agonist on nicotinic acetylcholine receptors believed to be at the heart of nicotine addiction. It was the first licensed smoking cessation drug (in the 1960s) and is widely available in some central and eastern European countries

Dependence: often used synonymously with 'addiction' but preferred in some quarters because of the stigma attached to 'addiction' (but see 'physical dependence')

Electronic cigarette (e-cigarette): a battery-powered device, sometimes looking similar to a cigarette, that aims to give much of the experience of smoking by using a heating element to vaporize a liquid containing nicotine. These devices are intended to deliver nicotine without the many toxins in cigarette smoke

Expired-air carbon monoxide: concentration of carbon monoxide (CO) – a product of incomplete combustion in cigarettes – in exhaled air; a value that gives an accurate index of CO in the blood and is used to measure the amount of cigarette smoke inhaled while smoking and to verify claims of abstinence (in which case the value should be less than 10 parts per million)

Half-life: time taken for the plasma concentration of an absorbed drug such as nicotine to decrease by 50% through elimination and metabolism

Nicotine: an alkaloid made by species of the tobacco plant; nicotine has psychological and physiological effects and typically causes dependence if ingested in a form that delivers it rapidly to the brain

Nicotine-replacement therapy (NRT): a medication that delivers pure nicotine into the bloodstream and thus helps smokers to stop smoking; the aim is to provide at least partial replacement, normally temporary, for the nicotine previously provided by cigarettes, with a view to easing cravings and symptoms of withdrawal and aiding smoking cessation

Nortriptyline: a tricyclic antidepressant found to be effective in aiding smoking cessation

Opportunistic advice: advice delivered by a health professional to a patient on the health professional's initiative

Physical dependence: physiological adaptation to a drug resulting in adverse symptoms ('withdrawal symptoms') when the drug is withdrawn

Varenicline: a partial agonist at the $\alpha_4\beta_2$ nicotinic receptor; licensed as an aid to smoking cessation (brand names Chantix, Champix)

Withdrawal syndrome: a constellation of temporary signs and symptoms caused by abstinence from a drug to which the body has become adapted

Introduction

Given the wide-ranging effects smoking has on many disease processes, it is essential that all clinicians understand:

- the short- and long-term effects of smoking on the body
- the benefits of smoking cessation
- why smokers find it difficult to stop
- the role of clinicians in promoting and supporting smoking cessation
- the treatments available to help smokers overcome their addiction.

Fast Facts: Smoking Cessation meets these needs: here, in one place, you will find all the information you need on smoking, tobacco addiction and how best to treat the addiction. As well as providing an evidence-based review of the social, psychological, economic and medical aspects of smoking addiction, we spell out the effects and consequences of smoking alongside the consequences of quitting.

The challenge for all of us is to make sure we give smokers the best opportunity and support to quit. Learn how to trigger more quit attempts, help patients overcome their addiction and improve long-term success using structured behavioral support and medications. With tips, advice and treatment aids for the clinical team, this up-to-date concise reference on everything to do with smoking and how to help smokers stop will benefit every clinician who comes into contact with smokers.

Ultimately, the best reason for reading this book is to help your patients who smoke to change their behavior for the better and sustainably. Success will result in a significant and wonderful improvement in people's health worldwide, and tremendous job satisfaction too.

The cigarette

There are many different varieties of cigarette tobacco, each with its own flavor and characteristics, and tobacco can be prepared in different ways that affect its taste, smell and pharmacological properties. Additives are included in cigarettes by the manufacturers to engineer an attractive and efficient nicotine delivery system. Table 1.1 lists some of the many thousands of chemicals in tobacco smoke.

One thing that all cigarettes have in common is that they deliver nicotine to the lungs. A puff on a cigarette results in rapid absorption of nicotine into the bloodstream and delivery of a high-concentration 'bolus' of nicotine to the brain by the arterial circulation (Figure 1.1); this process is repeated with every puff. In the UK and the USA, smokers absorb an average 1–2 mg of nicotine from each cigarette. This is only about

TABLE 1.1

Some of the substances a cigarette delivers into the body

- **Nicotine:** addictive; not carcinogenic; limited or no cardiovascular risk at doses typically obtained by smokers
- **Carbon monoxide:** reduces the blood's ability to carry oxygen; probably increases cardiovascular risk
- **Benzo(a)pyrene:** carcinogenic
- **Aromatic hydrocarbons:** carcinogenic
- **Nitrosamines:** carcinogenic
- **Additives:** enhance 'flavor' and nicotine effects
- **Particulates:** may carry acute risk of coronary thrombosis
- **Free radicals:** ionized particles may cause atherogenesis
- **Polonium:** radioactive element that may cause cancer

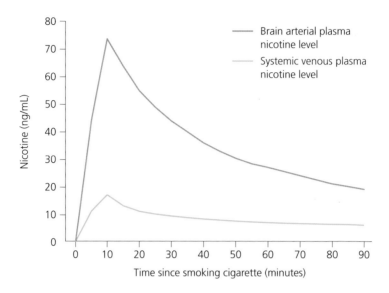

Figure 1.1 Concentrations of nicotine in brain arterial blood and systemic venous blood in a typical smoker following a single cigarette (the spike in arterial nicotine levels that occurs with each puff is not shown).

one-sixth to one-third of what they could obtain if they puffed more frequently and inhaled the smoke more deeply. In societies in which cigarettes are more expensive relative to earnings or in situations where cigarettes are otherwise not freely available, smokers take more nicotine from each cigarette, confirming that nicotine is the sought-after substance in tobacco.

Control of the nicotine dose. As a drug delivery system, cigarettes are very flexible because smokers can control the intensity and frequency of puffing. This 'fingertip control' of the nicotine dose allows smokers to meet their current need while avoiding the acute adverse effects of too much nicotine.

Many smokers, particularly older smokers and women, choose so-called 'light' or 'low-tar' brands, believing that these are safer. According to the reported analyses of their deliveries, these brands deliver as little as one-tenth of the tar and carbon monoxide of other brands. In fact, such reports are misleading:

the data are based on artificial measurements by smoking machines and do not mirror the actual delivery to a smoker. It is possible to extract as much tar and nicotine from these cigarettes as from higher-tar brands by more intensive puffing and by blocking the ventilation holes in the filter that would otherwise dilute the smoke – and that is exactly what smokers usually do. Each smoker appears to have a preferred level of nicotine intake and will adjust the way he or she smokes to achieve that level. Recognizing this, the terms 'light' and 'low tar' have been banned from cigarette packaging and marketing in the USA and EU.

Smokers who reduce the number of cigarettes they smoke typically compensate for the change by increasing the intensity of smoking such that smoke exposure remains unchanged. An exception is when they use another nicotine product at the same time, such as a nicotine patch or gum (see Chapter 7). It also appears that if cigarette consumption drops below a threshold (perhaps around 5 cigarettes per day), or if the cigarettes are designed to limit the potential for compensation (e.g. novel cigarettes in which the tobacco actually contains less nicotine), compensation is very limited.

Nicotine and its elimination from the body

Nicotine is an alkaloid obtained from tobacco plants and has wide-ranging effects on the central nervous system (CNS) (see pages 37–8). Its structure (Figure 1.2) resembles that of the major neurotransmitter acetylcholine, and it activates

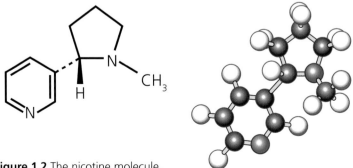

Figure 1.2 The nicotine molecule.

cholinergic receptors in the brain, which accounts for many of the psychoactive effects.

Once in the bloodstream, nicotine is distributed around the body, readily crossing cell membranes and entering every tissue. It is eliminated quite rapidly, mainly through metabolism, but partly by excretion in urine. It is metabolized mostly to the oxides cotinine and nicotine-1′-N-oxide. These appear to be largely inactive and are further metabolized and excreted in urine. The plasma concentration of nicotine reduces by half every 90–120 minutes (its half-life; see Figure 1.1).

Duration of withdrawal symptoms. All nicotine is cleared from the body within a day or two of abstinence. Some people think that this must therefore be the period when smokers experience withdrawal symptoms (see Chapter 5). However, the duration of withdrawal symptoms has nothing to do with this; it is related to how long it takes the body to get used to not having nicotine in the system. The duration for most symptoms is 2–4 weeks.

Estimating nicotine intake. Nicotine concentrations in the blood could conceptually be a useful index of dependence, but its short half-life means that a single measure does not give a particularly accurate picture of total intake over a day. Measurement of its metabolite, cotinine, is used instead. Cotinine has a half-life of 14–20 hours, so its concentration in the blood is more stable than that of nicotine and it can be easily measured in saliva, urine or even hair. Saliva samples are simple to obtain by means of a dental swab and are the method of choice for accurate estimation of daily nicotine intake.

A daily nicotine intake of 16 mg (approximately 16 cigarettes/ day, or one every hour) corresponds on average to a saliva cotinine concentration of 200 ng/mL; a daily nicotine intake of 10 mg generates a saliva cotinine concentration of about 125 ng/mL. These estimations are not the same for urine or blood measurements.

Monoamine oxidase inhibitors in cigarette smoke

There is evidence that cigarette smoke contains other psychoactive compounds which some now believe may contribute to its addictive properties. Most notably, there is at least one monoamine oxidase inhibitor (MAOI). MAOIs reduce the rate at which monoamine neurotransmitters such as dopamine are broken down and have been found to reduce depressive symptoms. In the case of smoking, they might contribute to the rewarding effect of cigarette smoke or act synergistically with nicotine (which is primarily rewarding as it causes release of dopamine in the nucleus accumbens – see Chapter 5). This may help explain why people who suffer from depression are particularly likely to smoke.

Research is in its early days, but if MAOIs play a role in cigarette addiction, pure nicotine delivery systems may be less addictive, even if they deliver nicotine as rapidly as cigarettes.

Key points – cigarettes as a nicotine delivery system

- Cigarettes deliver a 'bolus' of nicotine to the brain within seconds of each puff.
- Smokers absorb an average 1–2 mg of nicotine per cigarette (more when cigarettes are smoked more intensively).
- Cigarettes also deliver tar, containing potent carcinogens, and carbon monoxide.
- Smokers' intake of tar and nicotine from so-called 'low-tar' cigarettes is not substantially lower than the intake from higher-tar cigarettes.
- Nicotine is rapidly metabolized and excreted; its concentration in the blood halves every 90–120 minutes. Almost all the nicotine is cleared over a day of abstinence.
- The nicotine metabolite cotinine is eliminated much more slowly and is present in all body fluids, including saliva and urine; measurement of saliva or urine cotinine content is therefore a useful means of assessing total nicotine intake over the past few days.

Key references

Benowitz NL. Nicotine addiction. *N Engl J Med* 2010;2295–303.

Benowitz NL, Jacob P 3rd. Metabolism of nicotine to cotinine studied by a dual stable isotope method. *Clin Pharmacol Ther* 1994;56:483–93.

Nicotine Addiction in Britain – a Report of the Tobacco Advisory Group. London: Royal College of Physicians, 2000.

Prevalence

Geographic variation. The prevalence of cigarette smoking varies from country to country, as do rates for men and women (Figure 2.1).

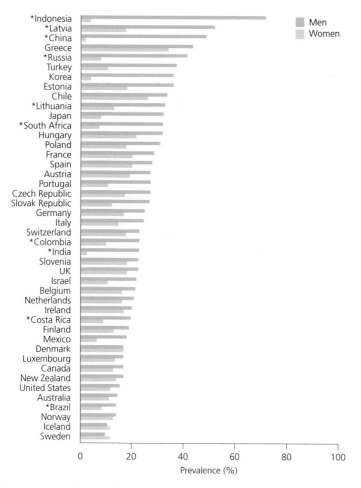

Figure 2.1 Prevalence of daily smokers, aged 15+, in 2013 (or nearest year).
*Non-OECD countries. Adapted from data from OECD Health Statistics 2014.

In countries such as the UK and the USA, rates are relatively low overall, and rates for women are slightly lower than those for men. However, in Asian and African countries the prevalence of smoking is much higher in men than in women.

Socioeconomic factors. Within countries, smoking prevalence varies according to socioeconomic status and level of education. In high-income countries such as the UK and the USA, smoking rates are higher among less affluent and less well-educated groups. Figure 2.2 shows the trends in Australia, and the pattern is similar in the UK and USA.

In the UK, the main cause of the socioeconomic gradient in smoking prevalence is a difference in the success of attempts to stop smoking. Thus, low-income smokers make the same number of quit attempts and want to stop just as much as higher-income smokers, but they are less likely to succeed. In other countries, different patterns may hold true.

Ethnic differences in smoking prevalence are often accompanied by sex differences. In general, women from Asian backgrounds are

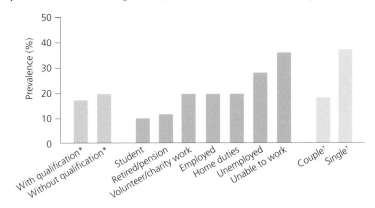

Figure 2.2 Prevalence of regular smokers in Australia as a function of educational level, employment status and household composition. *Post-school qualification. †With dependent children. Adapted from data from National Drug Strategy Household Survey, 2010, Australian Institute of Health and Welfare.

subject to strong cultural taboos against smoking, so that prevalence in women is much lower than in men. Among British Asians, smoking prevalence is highest in those of Bangladeshi descent, moderate in those of Pakistani descent and low in those of Indian descent. In the UK, there is also a high prevalence of smoking in people of African-Caribbean descent. In the USA, native American communities have particularly high smoking rates (Figure 2.3).

Changes in smoking prevalence. In many developed countries, smoking prevalence has fallen dramatically from a peak in the middle of the last century. At that time, most of the population smoked, whereas prevalence is now 20–30%. Figure 2.4 shows the decrease in smoking in men and women in Japan, the UK and the USA since the 1960s.

It is widely thought that it will become increasingly difficult to reduce smoking prevalence in countries such as the USA and UK as the persisting smokers will be more 'hard core'.

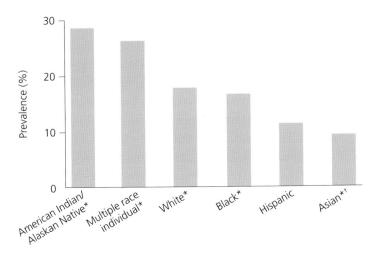

Figure 2.3 Prevalence of cigarette smoking in different ethnic groups in the USA. *Non-Hispanic. †In the USA, most Asians originate from the Far East, whereas British Asians are mainly descended from immigrants from the Indian subcontinent. Adapted from 2014 data from the US Centers for Disease Control and Prevention; Jamal A et al. 2015.

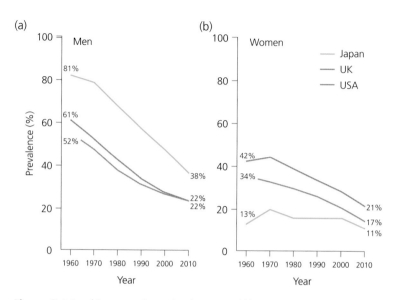

Figure 2.4 Smoking prevalence in a) men and b) women in Japan, the UK and the USA 1960–2010 (or latest available). Adapted from Eriksen M et al. *The Tobacco Atlas,* 4th edn. American Cancer Society, 2012.

However, this is not generally the case. The decline in the UK, averaged across men and women, has continued at the same pace since the 1970s (with a hiatus in the mid-1990s when there was minimal tobacco control activity). Moreover, as the prevalence of smoking has dropped, so has the daily cigarette consumption of the remaining smokers.

The commonly held view in the UK and the USA that women are more likely to smoke than men is unfounded. Not only do men continue to be more likely to smoke than women, but the difference is larger than it appears, because pipes and cigars, which are smoked almost exclusively by men, are not included in these figures – these would add about 2% to smoking prevalence in men. In addition, male smokers tend to smoke more heavily than female smokers.

In some other countries there is evidence of an increase, rather than a decrease, in smoking prevalence, as tobacco companies expand their markets. For example, prevalence seems to be rising in some countries in Eastern Europe. France has pulled back from strong anti-tobacco policies and this has been reflected by an increase in smoking rates.

Daily smoking patterns

The majority of smokers smoke every day. In England, just under 90% of smokers smoke daily. In the USA, the proportion of non-daily smokers has increased to around 25%, and is highest in states with the lowest smoking prevalence and most active tobacco control policies. The application of regulations that prevent smoking in indoor public areas may partly account for this increase, but there are probably other factors as well, including the changing social acceptability of smoking.

It should be noted that non-daily smokers do take in substantial amounts of nicotine – and probably, therefore, tobacco-related toxins from smoking. Further, non-daily smoking confers substantial health risks, especially from cardiovascular diseases. It is therefore misleading to report only daily smoking in the headline prevalence figures as is done in some countries such as Australia.

About 70% of smokers smoke their first cigarette of the day within 30 minutes of waking, relating to a high propensity to 'nicotine hunger' (cigarette addiction, as discussed in more detail in Chapter 5).

Starting to smoke

In the USA and the UK, people most commonly start smoking at 13–16 years of age. The reasons why young people become smokers are complex. Peer influence certainly plays a role and it is possible, though not established, that more distant role models (e.g. music and movie stars) may have an effect too. Personal characteristics are also important. In many western countries, those with an antisocial personality and/or lacking engagement with social values are more likely to take up smoking, as are those with a tendency toward sensation- or thrill-seeking (a characteristic common in teenagers). There is also evidence that children who suffer from depression are more likely to begin smoking, but the reverse is also true – non-depressed children who start to smoke are more likely to become depressed subsequently. This suggests that there may be a causal link in both directions, or that there is a common underlying mechanism.

Evidence on the influence of parental smoking is not as clear as one might expect. Some research has suggested that the influence is not one of direct role models, but may be related to a permissive attitude to smoking. However, there is also evidence that becoming a regular smoker is linked to a genetic susceptibility. The heritability of take-up of regular smoking in western countries has been put at around 50%. This statistic is comparable to that for alcoholism.

Attitudes to smoking and beliefs about the risks and benefits of smoking are quite closely linked to smoking behavior in young people, but, interestingly, are not particularly useful as predictors of smoking uptake. This suggests that either these attitudes and beliefs have little causal influence but, rather, fall into line with the behavior once it has started, or there is a rapid change just before the onset of smoking behavior. There may be a critical period during early adolescence when new attitudes and motivations are forming, which could in theory be targeted by social interventions aimed at reducing smoking uptake.

Smokers' attitudes and attempts to stop smoking

Surveys in Europe and the USA consistently show that the majority of smokers would like to stop. Approximately 80% have made at least one attempt to do so, and 30–50% make at least one attempt in any given year.

The main reasons for wanting to stop are shown in Table 2.1. At the top of the list in both the USA and the UK are concerns about health and the cost of cigarettes. Some smokers report that pressure from their children or spouse is a factor in the decision to try to stop.

TABLE 2.1

Common reasons for wanting to stop smoking

- Current health
- Worries about future health
- Cost of smoking
- Pressure from family
- Doctor's advice

Other forms of tobacco use

Although the focus of this book is on cigarette smoking, it must be remembered that pipe and cigar smoking present similar health risks if the smoke is inhaled. In both the USA and the UK about 2% of men smoke pipes or cigars, but not cigarettes.

Tobacco is also used in various 'smokeless' forms, including chewing tobacco, oral snuff (wads of tobacco placed between the gums and cheek) and nasal snuff (fine-ground tobacco that is sniffed into the nose). Use of smokeless tobacco products is common among certain sections of society in the USA, among Asian populations and in Sweden. Although the health risks from smokeless tobacco are substantially lower than those from smoking, they may nevertheless be significant. Oral cancers and possibly cardiovascular disease are of particular concern. It should be noted, however, that for certain forms of smokeless tobacco, such as Swedish 'snus' (coarse-ground unfermented tobacco and additives held as a wad in the mouth), there is little direct evidence for an increased risk of serious illnesses. This is because these forms contain only low levels of tobacco carcinogens.

Key points – smoking patterns

- Smoking prevalence varies across countries from less than 20% to more than 60% in men, and from less than 5% to more than 30% in women.
- Smoking prevalence is higher in men than in women in almost every country.
- In industrialized English-speaking countries (which have all implemented tobacco control measures), smoking prevalence has declined markedly, and in countries such as the UK and Australia with strong anti-tobacco policies it continues to decline.
- In western industrialized countries, smoking prevalence is greater among people with lower educational level and greater socioeconomic disadvantage.
- Most smokers smoke every day, and in the USA and the UK 70% smoke within 30 minutes of waking.
- Most smokers start during adolescence; initial take-up and transition to regular smoking are linked to both genetic and social factors.
- In most developed countries, most smokers want to stop smoking, usually because of health concerns and cost, and try to do so many times.

Key references

Australian Institute of Health and Welfare. Canberra: *2010 National Drug Strategy Household Survey Report*, July 2011. Drug Statistics Series Number 25.

Burt RD, Dinh KT, Peterson AV Jr, Sarason IG. Predicting adolescent smoking: a prospective study of personality variables. *Prev Med* 2000;30:115–25.

Castrucci BC, Gerlach KK, Kaufman NJ, Orleans CT. The association among adolescents' tobacco use, their beliefs and attitudes, and friends' and parents' opinions of smoking. *Matern Child Health J* 2002;6:159–67.

Centers for Disease Control and Prevention. *Current Cigarette Smoking Among U.S. Adults Aged 18 Years and Older*. www.cdc.gov/tobacco/campaign/tips/resources/data/cigarette-smoking-in-united-states.html, last accessed 29 February 2016.

Derzon JH, Lipsey MW. Predicting tobacco use to age 18: a synthesis of longitudinal research. *Addiction* 1999;94:995–1006.

Engels RC, Knibbe RA, Drop MJ. Predictability of smoking in adolescence: between optimism and pessimism. *Addiction* 1999;94:115–24.

Eriksen M, Mackay J, Schluger N et al. *The Tobacco Atlas*, 5th edn. The American Cancer Society and World Lung Foundation, 2015. www.tobaccoatlas.org, last accessed 29 February 2016.

Hall W, Madden P, Lynskey M. The genetics of tobacco use: methods, findings and policy implications. *Tob Control* 2002;11:119–24.

Jamal A, Homa DM, O'Connor E et al. Current cigarette smoking among adults – United States, 2005–2014. Centers for Disease Control and Prevention. *Morbidity and Mortality Weekly Report* 2015;64:1233–40.

Nicotine Addiction in Britain – a Report of the Tobacco Advisory Group. London: Royal College of Physicians, 2000.

OECD Health Statistics. *Non-Medical Determinants of Health: Tobacco Consumption*. http://stats.oecd.org, last accessed 29 February 2016.

Smith SS, Fiore MC. The epidemiology of tobacco use, dependence, and cessation in the United States. *Prim Care* 1999;26:433–61.

Tobacco in Australia. Facts and Issues. 1.7 *Trends in the prevalence of smoking by socioeconomic status*. www.tobaccoinaustralia.org.au/1-7-trends-in-the-prevalence-of-smoking-by-socioeconomic-status, last accessed 30 November 2015.

West R, McEwen A, Bolling K, Owen L. Smoking cessation and smoking patterns in the general population: a 1-year follow-up. *Addiction* 2001;96:891–902.

World Health Organization. *World Health Report 2002*. Geneva: WHO, 2002.

3 Social, psychological and economic influences on smoking

Social norms

Cigarette smoking is markedly influenced by social norms and other environmental influences. In cultures in which smoking is taboo for women, few women smoke.

Smoking prevalence has declined as smoking has become more marginalized in sections of western society. The influence of social norms is also manifest in regional variations in smoking prevalence within countries. In the UK, for example, smoking prevalence increases with 'northerliness', even controlling for social class.

Psychiatric disorders

There is a strong link between smoking and many psychiatric disorders, including mood disorders, schizophrenia and substance abuse. Smoking is also prevalent among homeless people, many of whom suffer from mental health disorders. Not only are persons with psychiatric disorders more likely to smoke, but they are also likely to smoke more heavily than others. It has yet to be established why these links exist: whether smoking causes or exacerbates these conditions, whether a disorder makes it more likely that a patient will smoke and be unable to stop, or whether there is a common underlying cause.

It is widely thought that smoking is particularly closely linked to schizophrenia, but in fact the dominant factors are the severity of the psychiatric disorder and whether the patient is institutionalized (Figure 3.1). Thus, discussion about whether specific links exist between smoking behavior and the mechanisms that underlie schizophrenia or its treatment are somewhat premature.

It is, however, clear that there is no evidence for deterioration overall in mental health when people with psychiatric disorders stop smoking and in some cases there may be an improvement.

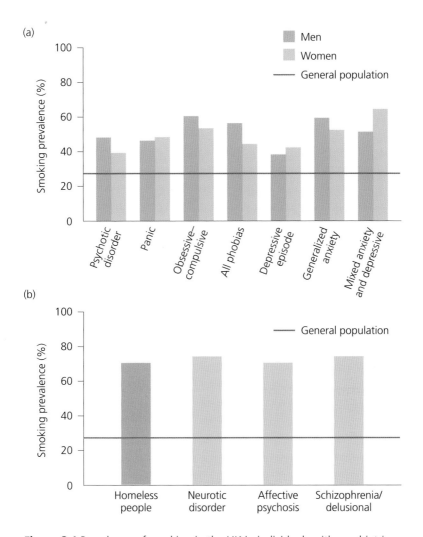

Figure 3.1 Prevalence of smoking in the UK in individuals with psychiatric disorders (the horizontal line represents smoking prevalence in the general adult population): (a) non-institutionalized patients; (b) institutionalized patients (and homeless persons for comparison). Data: Meltzer 1995 (Crown copyright material is reproduced with the permission of the Controller of HMSO and the Queen's Printer for Scotland).

Alcohol intake and other drug-related disorders

Smokers are particularly likely to experience problems with illicit psychoactive drugs and alcohol. The link with alcohol abuse and alcoholism is particularly strong, leading some to suggest that heavy smokers should be screened for alcoholism. Similarly, although drug abuse is rare in an absolute sense, smokers, especially heavy smokers, are far more likely than non-smokers to engage in drug abuse.

Smokers with alcohol use disorder find it harder to stop smoking; if they do stop, it does not adversely affect their prospects of recovery from that disorder, and may improve it.

Criminality and antisocial behavior

Adolescents who engage in antisocial behavior, truant from school and express antisocial attitudes are more likely to smoke than those who do not engage in antisocial behavior. In adulthood, there is a strong correlation between having a criminal conviction and being a smoker.

Government actions

Probably the greatest impact on smoking prevalence can be achieved through large-scale social and governmental policies. Table 3.1 summarizes the options and their likely effects.

Taxation is the most clearly established of the many ways in which governments can influence smoking. A 10% increase in the price of cigarettes relative to earnings is linked, on average, to a 4% reduction in consumption by adults. In teenagers, the effect is greater, with a 10% increase in cost linked to a 10% decrease in consumption.

In countries such as the UK, smokers support these kinds of policies, presumably because they recognize that they can provide an added incentive to stop – which is what they mostly want to do.

Taxation has to be linked to effective countermeasures against illicit supply. It is important to structure it to prevent

TABLE 3.1

Large-scale policies that can affect smoking prevalence

Increase in the price of cigarettes	On average, a 10% increase in real cost can lead to a 4% decrease in consumption
Mass media campaigns and events	Intensive and sustained campaigns and national quitting events increase smoking cessation rates and reduce smoking prevalence
Ban on advertising and promotion including brand imagery on packaging	Probably reduces smoking prevalence
Ban on smoking in indoor public areas	Appears to reduce smoking prevalence at least initially

tobacco companies using pricing policies to undermine its deterrent effect.

Not all of the decrease in consumption involves smokers giving up altogether; in some cases smokers merely reduce the number of cigarettes they smoke. The health benefits of this action may be undermined, however, because smokers tend to smoke each cigarette more intensively. It is also not fully known how reductions in consumption translate into health benefits. Nevertheless, it is clear that increasing the cost of smoking is, potentially, an important public health measure.

Mass media campaigns can be effective in promoting smoking cessation and reducing smoking prevalence. The size of the effect is related to the intensity of the campaign (as indexed by viewing numbers) and whether it is sustained. Specific quitting events, for example the UK's 'No Smoking Day' and 'Stoptober' (a mass quitting event that challenges smokers to be smoke-free for a month as a stepping stone to permanent cessation), and the US 'Great American Smokeout' (which encourages quitting for a day), have been evaluated as a highly cost-effective way of promoting smoking cessation.

Bans on tobacco advertising. Tobacco companies spend many billions of dollars annually promoting their brands. In many countries, including the USA, tobacco advertising is banned from television but is permitted in print media.

Where there have been more comprehensive bans on promotion, there has been some evidence of an effect in reducing smoking. For this reason, and because of moral concerns over permitting promotion of a product that is addictive and often lethal when used as intended, several countries, including those in the European Union, have implemented a total ban on tobacco promotion. An international treaty, the Framework Convention on Tobacco Control (see Chapter 8) mandates this and other tobacco control measures.

Plain packaging. Several countries have implemented legislation requiring cigarette and tobacco to be sold in standard plain packages carrying graphic health warnings and the brand name in a standard font with no brand imagery. The effect is expected primarily to be on take-up of smoking – with cigarettes becoming less attractive to adolescents.

Indoor smoking bans have been introduced in public indoor areas in many countries, including the UK, Australia and New Zealand, and in most jurisdictions in the USA. Although the bans were introduced to protect the health of non-smokers, there is some evidence that they might have at least a short-term effect in reducing smoking prevalence.

Key points – social, psychological and economic influences on smoking

- In western countries, smoking is more prevalent in people with mental health problems, those with alcohol- and drug-related problems, the homeless and criminals.
- Smoking prevalence is strongly influenced by social norms and the financial cost. High-intensity and sustained mass media campaigns and mass quitting events, such as Stoptober, have an important effect in promoting smoking cessation and reducing smoking prevalence. Banning tobacco marketing and bans on smoking in indoor public areas probably also play a role.

Key references

Action on Smoking and Health. *All Party Parliamentary Group on Smoking and Health. Inquiry into the Effectiveness and Cost-effectiveness of Tobacco Control.* London: ASH, 2010. www.ash.org.uk/files/documents/ASH_743.pdf, last accessed 29 February 2016.

Lawrence D, Mitrou F, Zubrick SR. Smoking and mental illness: results from population surveys in Australia and the United States. *BMC Public Health* 2009;9:285.

McManus S, Meltzer H, Campion H. *Cigarette smoking and mental health in England. Data from the Adult Psychiatric Morbidity Survey 2007.* National Centre for Social Research, December 2010. www.natcen.ac.uk/media/21994/smoking-mental-health.pdf, last accessed 29 February 2016.

Meltzer H. *OPCS Surveys of Psychiatric Morbidity in Great Britain Report 1: The Prevalence of Psychiatric Morbidity among Adults Living in Private Households.* London: HMSO, 1995.

Tobacco Advisory Group. *Nicotine Addiction in Britain – a Report of the Tobacco Advisory Group.* London: Royal College of Physicians, 2000.

4 Effects of smoking and smoking cessation

Early smoking experiences

The irritancy of nicotine and other components of smoke in the airways usually causes coughing and sore throat on initial exposure. For many people this is accompanied by nausea and dizziness caused by the action of nicotine on the central nervous system (CNS) and by the anoxic effect of inhaling carbon monoxide. There may also be a sensation of cooling in the hands and feet, palpitations, sweating and tremor. Some first-time smokers experience a pleasurable sensation as well. Adaptation to the acute unpleasant effects of smoking occurs quickly, and within a few weeks or months novice smokers are able to tolerate as much nicotine from each cigarette as habitual smokers.

Long-term health effects of smoking

Long-term smoking has disastrous effects on most body systems, resulting in the death of half of smokers who do not manage to stop (Table 4.1); it kills an estimated 6 million people worldwide each year. Those who are killed by smoking die an average of 20 years sooner than they would have done otherwise. Smoking also causes long-term disability, both in those who are eventually killed by cigarette smoking and in those who ultimately die from some other cause. The average smoker who fails to stop can expect to develop diseases of old age many years earlier than a non-smoker. The following sections discuss some of the more common causes of death associated with smoking.

Lung cancer kills about 150 000 people a year in the USA and 30 000 in the UK. Although a variety of new techniques are being tested to detect lung cancer in its early stages, in practice the disease is usually fatal. Smoking accounts for the vast

TABLE 4.1

Deaths attributable to smoking*

Cause	Men (%)	Women (%)
Cancers		
Trachea, lung, bronchus	87	73
Larynx	81	74
Upper respiratory sites	72	49
Esophagus	68	60
Bladder	43	28
Kidney and renal pelvis	33	8
Stomach	25	11
Pancreas	23	24
Myeloid leukemia	22	9
Cervical	–	11
Unspecified site	53	21
Respiratory		
COPD	88	81
Chronic airway obstruction	78	76
Pneumonia, influenza	23	14
Heart and circulation		
Aortic aneurysm	62	55
Atherosclerosis	27	12
Other heart disease	18	10
Other arterial disease	17	18
Ischemic heart disease	15	10
Cerebrovascular disease	13	6
Others		
Stomach/duodenal ulcer	52	45

*Registered deaths among adults aged 35 and over in England, as a percentage of all deaths from that disease. COPD, chronic obstructive pulmonary disease.

Source: *Statistics on Smoking: England 2014.* Health and Social Care Information Centre, October 2014. www.hscic.gov.uk/catalogue/PUB14988/ smok-eng-2014-rep.pdf, last accessed 29 February 2016.

majority of cases of lung cancer worldwide. Indeed, lung cancer was almost never seen before manufactured cigarettes became popular at the beginning of the 1900s. Since then, it has reached epidemic proportions. The risk of lung cancer is 15 times greater for a smoker than for a non-smoker. The risk accumulates over time and is related to both daily cigarette consumption and duration of smoking. Starting young – before 15 years of age – is particularly hazardous. About 1 in 8 smokers who do not quit will die from lung cancer.

There are two major types of lung cancer: small-cell lung cancer (SCLC) and non-small-cell lung cancer (NSCLC, including squamous-cell carcinoma, adenocarcinoma and large-cell carcinoma). Both are usually caused by smoking. NSCLC is much more common, accounting for about 80% of all cases, and usually spreads to other parts of the body more slowly than SCLC.

Cardiovascular disease is the leading cause of death and a major cause of long-term disability in western societies. It includes coronary artery disease (stable and unstable angina, acute myocardial infarction and sudden death), cerebrovascular disease (cerebral infarction and cerebral and subarachnoid hemorrhage), peripheral arterial disease (large and small vessel) and aortic aneurysm.

Smoking can cause both acute and chronic cardiac and vascular events by a wide variety of mechanisms – hematologic, neurohormonal, metabolic, hemodynamic, molecular, genetic and biochemical. The average middle-aged smoker's risk of contracting heart disease in a 10-year period is approximately double that of someone who has never smoked. Unlike the risk for lung cancer, cardiovascular risk is not directly proportional to overall smoke exposure. Approximately half the increased risk occurs even with very light smoking, and the risk curve flattens somewhat above about 10 cigarettes per day. Even non-daily smokers incur significant cardiovascular risk. This probably reflects the acute increase in risk of myocardial infarction on inhalation of smoke particles, independent of the length of the smoking history; the remainder of the excess risk arises from long-term damage to the vascular system. Recent research has found that smoking as few as three cigarettes per day increases the risk of heart attack.

The cardiovascular effects of acute exposure to even small amounts of cigarette smoke likely account for some of the adverse effects on non-smokers exposed to cigarette smoke. Multiple studies have shown immediate and dramatic drops in heart attacks among non-smokers when smoking is banned in public places.

Chronic obstructive pulmonary disease (COPD) is, like lung cancer, relatively uncommon in non-smokers in western countries. However, it is easier to detect at an earlier stage (although patients often present at a late stage when symptoms are significantly effecting their lifestyle), and its progress can be stopped though not reversed. The only truly effective course of action is to stop smoking, but most patients with COPD, even those with advanced disease, have considerable difficulty with this.

The term COPD encompasses chronic bronchitis and emphysema. In both disorders, the lungs lose their ability to transfer oxygen to the bloodstream, and so the person is, in effect, asphyxiating. In the case of chronic bronchitis, the smoker develops a chronic cough that gradually worsens over a period of years. In emphysema, the lungs lose their elasticity, and the patient cannot draw sufficient breath. In both cases, the smoker finds that he or she becomes breathless with the slightest exertion and, as the disease progresses, the smoker experiences 'exacerbations' – bouts of serious respiratory distress in which breathing becomes extremely difficult. Eventually, the smoker dies from one of these exacerbations or experiences complications from the chronic breathing problems.

COPD is progressive and can be detected by observing the change over time in the results of a simple lung function test such as the FEV_1 (the forced expiratory volume in 1 second, or maximum amount of air that can be exhaled in 1 second). If this is measured regularly (yearly), the rate of decline can be compared with that expected as a consequence of normal aging. This approach, together with a vigorous and intensive smoking cessation program, has been found to be an effective means of encouraging quitting in a substantial number of smokers.

For more information on COPD see *Fast Facts: Chronic Obstructive Pulmonary Disease*.

Other life-threatening diseases. Smoking is linked to a large number of cancers (see Table 4.1), including many in organs that do not come into direct contact with cigarette smoke, such as the bladder. This is because the carcinogens in cigarette smoke are absorbed and distributed throughout the body, where they can affect susceptible tissues.

Smoking is also linked to gastric ulcers and circulatory diseases, which lead to death in considerable numbers of patients, and to suffering and disability in many more. Even now, science is discovering new contributions that smoking makes to diseases not initially considered related to smoking.

There was a view in the 1990s that smoking was protective against Alzheimer's disease. We now know that smoking is an important risk factor for both Alzheimer's and non-Alzheimer's dementia.

Non-life-threatening diseases. The number of disorders known to be linked to smoking is growing. Those that have been discovered to date are listed in Table 4.2. Some of these are quite well known to smokers whereas others, such as macular degeneration – causing blindness – and age-related hearing loss, will be surprising to many people.

Smoking can also have an effect on various treatment regimens or medical conditions. Some common examples are given in Table 4.3. It is useful for clinicians to be aware of these links.

TABLE 4.2

Non-life-threatening physical diseases linked to smoking

- Age-related hearing loss
- Cataract
- Cold injuries (tissue damage caused by exposure to cold environment)
- Crohn's disease
- Diabetes mellitus (type 2)
- Erectile dysfunction
- Gum disease
- Macular degeneration
- Osteoarthritis
- Osteoporosis
- Rheumatoid arthritis
- Skin wrinkles

Smoking and reproduction

It is widely known that maternal smoking during pregnancy reduces birth weight. This effect is partly due to increased risk of premature labor and partly because babies are small for their gestational age. Many pregnant smokers and even some clinicians fail to appreciate the significance of this low birth weight: it is directly linked to an increased risk of stillbirth and death for the baby during childbirth or soon afterwards. There is also some evidence that low birth weight is linked to an increased risk of cardiovascular and lung disease in the offspring in middle age. The mechanism linking smoking with these consequences has not been clearly established. It could in part be related to the influence of carbon monoxide on placental oxygen transfer, but nicotine may also play a role.

Fertility is impaired by smoking in both women and men. Smoking is also an important cause of miscarriage, the risk being

35

TABLE 4.3

Effect of smoking on medical treatments

Treatment	Effects and notes
Insulin	• Risks caused by smoking and diabetes are synergistic • Smokers may not know the risks, and should be made fully aware of them • Smoking affects insulin response, so insulin dose may need to be changed if smoker stops
General anesthesia	• Smokers require more careful management and may need different doses of anesthetic agents • Most smokers are not aware of their increased risk under anesthesia; counseling by the anesthetist leads some to stop smoking
Surgical healing	• Wound healing is slower in smokers than in non-smokers; smokers are more vulnerable to complications from surgery • Smokers should be encouraged to stop smoking as early as possible before surgery
Fertility treatment	• Smokers have a markedly reduced response to fertility treatment • Many smokers are not aware of this; all smoking patients (male and female) should be advised that they are hampering their chances of conceiving and should be strongly urged to stop smoking

several times higher than in non-smokers when other known risk factors are controlled for. In addition, smoking increases the risk of placental abruption (in which the placenta detaches from the wall of the uterus), which jeopardizes the lives of both the baby and the mother. It is important for pregnant smokers to understand that, even if the baby is born apparently healthy, this does not mean that no damage has been done. Children of smokers are more likely to suffer from intellectual impairment and behavioral problems and delinquency, although we cannot be sure that smoking is the cause. Also, there is evidence that smoking (and possibly any form of nicotine use) during pregnancy increases the subsequent risk of sudden infant death syndrome (crib or cot death).

Effects of nicotine

At the doses absorbed by smokers, nicotine is not known to cause major physical illness, except in certain categories of patient, for example those susceptible to Buerger's syndrome, in which circulation to the limbs is lost, and possibly in pregnancy. Nicotine does not cause cancer. The main effects of nicotine are on the autonomic nervous systems and CNS and are caused by its action at synapses. Nicotine binds to a particular family of acetylcholine (ACh) receptors known as the nicotinic ACh receptors and in many cases increases the activity in the neural pathways concerned, at least initially.

In the autonomic nervous system, nicotine acts primarily as a stimulant. Acutely, it raises heart rate and blood pressure, constricts capillaries in the extremities and causes tremor and sweating. Larger doses produce larger effects. At very high concentrations (beyond those normally seen in smokers) nicotine blocks peripheral ACh receptors, leading to muscle rigidity and paralysis.

In the brain, nicotine has a wide range of both acute and chronic effects. At smoking doses it initially increases ACh release in the cortex and dopamine release in the nucleus accumbens. Subsequently, it desensitizes or inactivates nicotine receptors in the brain. This action is believed to play an important role in the addictive potential of nicotine (see Chapter 5).

Long-term nicotine ingestion results in an increase in the number of certain types of nicotinic ACh receptors in the brain. The functional significance of this is not clear. Recent evidence indicates that it is not the underlying reason for cigarette craving, because non-addictive drugs such as varenicline also lead to this increase.

Until recently it was thought that ingesting as little as 60 mg nicotine would be fatal to an adult. However, it turns out that this arose from an unreliable historical source. The fatal dose is probably much higher and nicotine ingested orally typically induces vomiting at doses much lower than lethal doses, which limits the risk of long-term damage.

Acute effects of stopping smoking

When smokers abstain, even for a few hours, they experience physical and psychological changes, most of which are unpleasant (Table 4.4). Most or all are attributable to cessation of nicotine intake. However, not all of them should be regarded as part of a withdrawal syndrome. Such a syndrome involves signs and symptoms that arise when an individual abstains from a drug, because the body has adapted to the presence of the drug and needs a period of adjustment once the drug is no longer in the system. Thus, a key feature of a withdrawal syndrome is that it is temporary. While this is clearly the case for many of the subjective symptoms, such as depressed mood and irritability, it does not seem to be the case for some of the physical changes, which appear to be permanent and may simply reflect a return to a level that would have been the case if the individual had never smoked.

One such permanent change is the reduction in heart rate. Nicotine increases the heart rate acutely; it decreases again when nicotine is eliminated from the body. Another 'offset effect' is an increase in skin temperature. Nicotine causes the capillaries under the skin to constrict, thus reducing skin temperature. The temperature normalizes during abstinence. Smoking also leads to an increase in tremor, due to a nicotine-induced increase in sympathetic activation. When smokers abstain, the tremor reduces to normal.

One unpleasant and relatively long-lasting effect of abstinence is an increase in mouth ulcers. The cause is not known, and the effect is relatively uncommon, but when it occurs it can cause considerable discomfort. It is probably unrelated to nicotine.

TABLE 4.4

Acute effects of stopping smoking

Effect	Prevalence	Typical duration
Symptoms		
Irritability or aggression	> 25%	< 4 weeks
Increased appetite	> 25%	> 10 weeks
Difficulty concentrating	> 25%	< 4 weeks
Restlessness	> 25%	< 4 weeks
Depressed mood	< 25%	< 4 weeks
Urge to smoke	> 25%	> 10 weeks but declines
Sleep disturbance	< 25%	< 4 weeks
Signs		
Weight gain	> 25%	Permanent
Cough/sore throat	< 25%	< 4 weeks
Mouth ulcers	< 25%	> 2 weeks
Reduced heart rate	> 25%	Permanent
Reduced epinephrine (adrenaline) secretion	Unknown	< 2 weeks
Reduced cortisol secretion	Unknown	< 4 weeks
Increased skin temperature	> 25%	Permanent
Reduced tremor	> 25%	Permanent
Decreased sIgA secretion	> 25%	< 2 weeks
Increased slow-wave alpha activity on EEG	Unknown	Unknown

EEG, electroencephalogram; sIgA, secretory immunoglobulin A.
Adapted from Hughes et al. 1994.

Some smokers report coughs and sore throats when they stop smoking. Until recently this was regarded as nothing more than a sign of the cilia, which clear the lungs of mucus, becoming active again. However, it now appears that smokers have a genuinely increased susceptibility to upper respiratory tract infections or upper airways hypersensitivity for the first week or two after stopping. Any increased susceptibility to infection is probably linked to a short-term decrease in secretory immunoglobulin A in the saliva, which forms part of the body's defense mechanism. The reason for this decrease is not known.

Some smokers are very concerned about putting on weight if they quit smoking. It seems to deter many people from attempting to stop smoking. Clinicians may be tempted to reassure smokers that the gain in weight is temporary, but the evidence contradicts this. Weight gain is often progressive for a period of at least a year. The average weight gain in the first year is 6–8 kg. In a large clinical trial of smoking cessation, 33% of the ex-smokers gained more than 10 kg. The weight gain appears to represent more than just a return to the weight that smokers would have achieved had they never smoked; ex-smokers typically weigh more than those who have never smoked.

The core of the nicotine withdrawal syndrome is mood disturbance. The temporary mood changes that smokers experience when they stop are often unpleasant and disruptive; they have been compared with the effects of psychiatric disorders. Particular concern has been expressed about the increase in depressed mood, which has been linked in some studies (but not others) to subsequent relapse to smoking. However, there is no clear evidence that stopping smoking places smokers at greater risk of developing depression.

It is widely believed that smoking helps to relieve stress and anxiety, and that anxiety levels increase during abstinence. However, current evidence demonstrates that smoking does not actually help to reduce the stress. There is some evidence for a brief increase in anxiety when smokers stop smoking, but anxiety and stress levels soon fall to below their smoking level.

Many smokers report difficulty concentrating when they stop smoking, and objective tests confirm an observable decline in mental performance. This decline may interfere with work performance and with driving or operation of machinery, but is relatively short lived.

Health benefits of quitting

Quitting has substantial health benefits at any age. The greatest benefit is achieved in those who stop while they are relatively young, and before they develop a smoking-related disease, but all smokers stand to gain by quitting. In fact, a healthy adult who stops smoking before 35 years of age can have a near-normal life expectancy. Someone who stops in their forties or fifties can expect to gain an average of 6 years of healthy life.

Table 4.5 shows the main health benefits and how long they take to materialize. Every year after the age of about 35 years that a smoker delays smoking cessation costs an average of 2–3 months of life and *every day that smoking continues costs 4–6 hours of life expectancy.*

TABLE 4.5

Major health benefits of stopping smoking

Benefit within weeks

- Halts steep decline in lung function / reduces mortality from COPD
- Reduces postoperative complication rate
- Reduces risk of stillbirth, low birth weight in infants and complications of pregnancy
- Reduces risk of sudden death from cardiac event
- Reduces incidence of respiratory infections
- Reduces severity of asthma attacks
- Reduces age-related hearing loss
- Improves complexion

Benefits within a year

- Reduces risk of cardiovascular disease

Benefit after several years

- Halts rise in lung cancer risk
- Reduces risk of other cancers

COPD, chronic obstructive pulmonary disease.

One might expect that cessation of nicotine intake would result in a decrease in blood pressure, but this is not the case. Although a single dose of nicotine raises blood pressure in a non-smoker, it seems that adaptation occurs and smokers do not typically have higher blood pressure than non-smokers (controlling for other factors such as body mass index). Indeed, on rare occasions cessation of smoking has been found to be followed by an increase in blood pressure and even manifest hypertension. The reason for this is not clear.

Key points – effects of smoking and smoking cessation

- Smoking causes substantial mortality and morbidity, killing an estimated 6 million people worldwide each year.
- The main causes of death from smoking are lung cancer, cardiovascular disease and chronic obstructive pulmonary disease.
- Smoking also increases the risk of a wide range of disabling conditions, such as age-related blindness, deafness and dementia.
- Smoking impairs fertility and increases the risk of fetal and neonatal death.
- Stopping smoking reduces the risks; a healthy smoker who stops before 35 years of age has a near-normal life expectancy.
- Nicotine binds to nicotinic acetylcholine receptors and acts, among other things, as a central nervous system stimulant. Nicotine at the level associated with smoking has relatively few adverse health effects and does not cause cancer.
- Smoking cessation causes temporary withdrawal symptoms, such as irritability, restlessness, depressed mood, difficulty concentrating and increased appetite.
- Many smokers experience permanent weight gain when they stop smoking.

Key references

APA. *Diagnostic and Statistical Manual of Mental Disorders*, 4th edn. Washington, DC: American Psychiatric Association, 1995.

Benowitz NL. *Nicotine Safety and Toxicity.* Oxford: Oxford University Press, 1998.

Griesel AG, Germishuys PJ. Salivary immunoglobulin A levels of persons who have stopped smoking. *Oral Surg Oral Med Oral Pathol Oral Radiol Endod* 1999;87:170–3.

Hughes JR, Higgins ST, Bickel WK. Nicotine withdrawal versus other drug withdrawal syndromes: similarities and dissimilarities. *Addiction* 1994;89:1461–70.

MacNee W, Rennard SI. *Fast Facts: COPD*, 3rd edn. Oxford: Health Press, 2016.

O'Hara P, Connett JE, Lee WW et al. Early and late weight gain following smoking cessation in the Lung Health Study. *Am J Epidemiol* 1998;148:821–30.

Prescott E, Scharling H, Osler M, Schnohr P. Importance of light smoking and inhalation habits on risk of myocardial infarction and all cause mortality. A 22-year follow up of 12149 men and women in The Copenhagen City Heart Study. *J Epidemiol Community Health* 2002;56:702–6.

RCGP. *Nicotine Addiction in Britain – a Report of the Tobacco Advisory Group.* London: Royal College of Physicians, 2000.

Shannon-Cain J, Webster SF, Cain BS. Prevalence of and reasons for preoperative tobacco use. *AANA J* 2002;70:33–40.

USDHHS. *The Health Benefits of Smoking Cessation: A Report of the Surgeon General.* Rockville, MD: United States Department of Health and Human Services, 1990.

Ussher M, West R, McEwen A. Increases in cold symptoms and mouth ulcers on stopping smoking. *Tob Control* 2003;12:86–8.

West R. Smoking and pregnancy. *Fetal Maternal Med Rev* 2002;13:181–94.

What is addiction?

Drug addiction used to be thought of as a biological need for a drug that arises because of physiological adaptation to the presence of the drug in the body. The body becomes 'dependent' on the drug to be able to function normally. The brain adapts to exposure to the drug, so that when the drug is removed from the system, the brain enters a heightened state of excitability.

This 'physical dependence' model of addiction is no longer considered complete. A key problem now recognized is that the drug-taking and drug-seeking activities continue to be subject to powerful motivational forces that undermine and overwhelm attempts at restraint. In other words, the addict's whole motivational system is subverted by the drug creating powerful urges, desires or needs to engage in the drug-taking behavior despite the actual or potential harm being caused.

The way in which addiction is perceived has changed because the old version failed to capture the essence of the problem as it manifests itself clinically and socially. It is relatively straightforward to control the withdrawal symptoms with medication, or at least make the addict reasonably comfortable, during the transition period of 'detoxification'. However, in the great majority of cases, the addict returns to drug use later. The behavior is therefore clearly not determined solely by a need to avoid the withdrawal syndrome. In confirmation of this, research has shown that the severity of the withdrawal syndrome is not a consistently good predictor of relapse to drug use.

Thus, 'physical dependence' leading to a withdrawal syndrome plays a role, but it is far from the whole story. For all addictive drugs, the defining feature is that the behavior in question has come to dominate the addict's life in a way that is unwelcome and causes significant harm.

Mechanisms underlying cigarette addiction

There are almost certainly several mechanisms underlying smoking addiction, all involving nicotine in some way.

Habit. One likely mechanism involves the development of a powerful 'habit' in which cues associated with smoking trigger an urge to smoke. This occurs because nicotine acts on a part of the brain that learns which responses are useful for survival in different situations. This part of the brain evolved in other species and operates at a level below conscious awareness. Thus, smokers experience urges to smoke when confronted with smoking cues, but these need not stem from any anticipated pleasure from smoking or conscious decision-making process. The facilitation of such compelling associations probably requires nicotine to be delivered rapidly, as from a cigarette, rather than slowly as from, say, the nicotine patch.

The biological basis for this process centers on a neural pathway in the brain that runs from the ventral tegmental area (VTA) in the midbrain and ends in the nucleus accumbens in the forebrain (Figure 5.1).

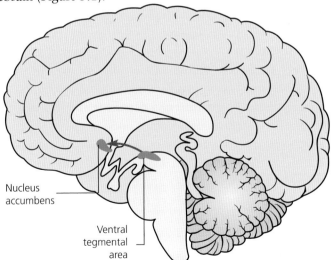

Nucleus accumbens

Ventral tegmental area

Figure 5.1 The central reward pathway (mesolimbic dopamine pathway) on which nicotine acts.

45

An initial rapid increase in the concentration of nicotine in the VTA leads to a burst of activity in the neurons in this pathway, leading to dopamine release in the nucleus accumbens. This dopamine release acts as a 'teaching signal', generating the impulse to smoke when the stimuli that preceded the dopamine release are encountered again.

Nicotine hunger. A second likely mechanism is the development of a kind of 'nicotine hunger'. Repeated intake of nicotine from cigarettes over a period of months or years changes the way that the pathway described above operates, so that if nicotine concentrations in the brain fall below a certain level, the activity in the pathway falls to abnormally low levels; this creates a kind of 'acquired drive', a hunger for nicotine, that is often experienced as craving. Like hunger for food, at low levels this feeling does not reach consciousness until something reminds us of its presence. At higher levels it is persistent and insistent, trying in some sense to motivate the smoker to do something to relieve it. It is a need.

Withdrawal symptoms. A third mechanism involves learning that smoking a cigarette helps to alleviate feelings of anxiety, depression, irritability, restlessness, and difficulty concentrating. These are all withdrawal symptoms resulting from physiological adaptation to repeated nicotine intake. Thus, nicotine does not alleviate these problems in people who do not smoke. Unfortunately, such discomfort can occur for all kinds of reasons, and the smoker's brain is not good at discriminating adverse mood states that arise from nicotine withdrawal from those arising from other causes. This means that smokers learn to associate adverse mood states and difficulty concentrating with smoking, and come to believe that smoking helps them to cope, even though it does so only because they are experiencing the problem because they have not smoked for a while. Unfortunately, as long as they believe that smoking helps to relieve adverse mood and other symptoms, smokers will be at risk of relapse when they try to stop.

The sum of motivations. Putting all this together, we can see that there are probably at least three ways in which repeated ultra-rapid intake of nicotine from cigarettes creates powerful motivations to smoke, which undermine and overwhelm the resolve not to. Different smokers probably experience each of these three elements of nicotine dependence to differing degrees. Thus, some smokers clearly have a strong nicotine hunger and smoke as soon as they wake up in the morning and whenever the opportunity arises during the day. Others may not need to smoke for much of the day but experience powerful urges to smoke in particular situations, such as when socializing; this is particularly true of non-daily smokers. For some smokers the nicotine withdrawal syndrome is relatively mild, while others experience severe adverse mood states when not smoking.

Of course, there is more to smoking than this: enjoyment of smoking, social rewards and attachment to the 'smoker identity' all play some role (Figure 5.2). Together they mean that smokers are often ambivalent about stopping, and when

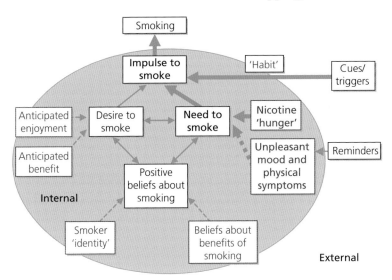

Figure 5.2 Sources of motivation to smoke. Thick arrows show pathways that directly involve nicotine dependence and are important in causing a return to smoking during attempts at abstinence.

they try, they find it very difficult – they are addicted to
cigarettes.

Recognizing an addicted smoker

Most smokers encountered by clinicians can be assumed to be
addicted to some degree. That is because they will be aware of
the health effects and in most cases have tried to stop at some
point in the past, usually many times. This does not mean that
they cannot stop, just that the more help they are given, the
better their chances of success.

Addicted smokers can be recognized or diagnosed in several
ways. A simple indicator of dependence is smoking soon after
waking. Because most nicotine is cleared overnight, smokers
wake in a state of nicotine deprivation, and those who act
quickly to replenish their nicotine levels are displaying their
dependence. In the USA and the UK, some 70% of smokers
light their first cigarette within 30 minutes of waking, and this
is often considered a marker of dependence.

Combining time to first cigarette of the day and number of
cigarettes smoked provides what is known as the Heaviness of
Smoking Index (HSI), which is probably the measure of choice
for very quickly assessing cigarette addiction (Table 5.1).

The diagnosis can also be made based on clinical evidence. If
a patient has tried to stop smoking and failed because the urge
to smoke is too strong, the need for a cigarette is overwhelming,
or the withdrawal symptoms are too much to bear, that patient
is addicted to cigarettes. Equally, if a patient has never tried to
stop smoking because the prospect of going without cigarettes
is too much to contemplate, even though he or she is concerned
about the damage that smoking is doing to his or her health,
that patient is addicted.

The fifth edition of the American Psychiatric Association's
Diagnostic and Statistical Manual of Mental Disorders (2013)
provides a set of formal criteria for 'drug dependence', which
are supposed to apply to smoking. Unfortunately, research
shows that these fail even the most basic test of a measure of

TABLE 5.1

The heaviness of smoking index

Use the following test to score a patient's level of nicotine dependence once they have been identified as a current or recent smoker

How soon after waking do you smoke your first cigarette?	
Within 5 minutes	3
5–30 minutes	2
31–60 minutes	1
60+ minutes	0

How many cigarettes a day do you smoke?	
10 or less	0
11–20	1
21–30	2
31 or more	3
	Total score

1–2, very low dependence; 3, low to moderate dependence; 4, moderate dependence; 5–6, high dependence.
Reproduced with permission from Kozlowski LT et al. 1994.

addiction to cigarettes – predicting relapse in people who try to stop smoking – so it is not recommended to use them.

Natural history of quitting

Given the strength of the physiological and behavioral forces driving continued smoking, it should not be surprising that quitting is difficult and the chances of success of any one attempt are low. Figure 5.3 depicts the 'survival curve' (in this case, the percentage who remain abstinent as time progresses) for a group of smokers quitting without medication or counseling. It shows that 75% of efforts fail within 1 week. By 12 months, more than 95% have relapsed. These outcomes

49

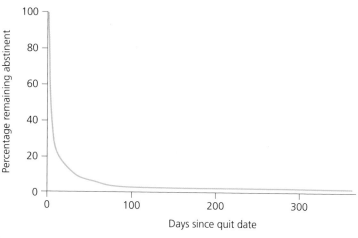

Figure 5.3 'Survival curve' showing the percentage of would-be quitters who remain abstinent in a typical unaided attempt to stop smoking.

parallel those seen in heroin addicts or alcoholics who try to achieve abstinence; fortunately, success rates can be improved by treatment, as discussed below.

As Figure 5.3 shows, the risk of relapse is greatest early on in the quit effort, with a sharp drop-off in the first week. After 2–3 months, the risk is considerably reduced, but even after abstaining for 6 months, smokers have about a 50% chance of eventually relapsing (Figure 5.4).

The process of relapse often starts with an initial episode involving very little smoking – as little as a puff or two – which the smoker may excuse as insignificant. Research shows, however, that smokers who smoke at all, even a puff, are extremely likely to relapse completely. This makes it imperative that smokers avoid any smoking, no matter how minor. These initial smoking episodes tend to happen – somewhat predictably – in circumstances in which the smoker is exposed to cues that elicit craving. Emotional upset, alcohol consumption and exposure to other smokers or other smoking cues are the three most common situations.

Emotional upset (whether the person is angry, miserable or anxious) may result in a lapse, perhaps because it is imagined

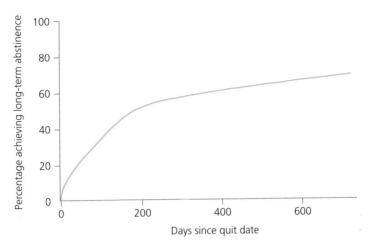

Figure 5.4 Likelihood of permanent success at stopping smoking having lasted for different periods of time in an unaided quit attempt.

that smoking will help with management of their emotional state. The fact that emotional upset undermines the person's ability and motivation to cope and exercise restraint is also important.

Alcohol consumption. Lapses are more likely when the smoker has been drinking, because smoking is associated with drinking and possibly because alcohol intoxication may undermine resolve.

Exposure to other smokers or other smoking cues. The sight and smell of smoking naturally prompts craving, and proximity to smokers means cigarettes are readily available.

Such cues can exert powerful effects: brain imaging studies have demonstrated specific patterns of brain activation when smokers are exposed to such cues. Furthermore, behavioral studies have shown that smokers in the grip of a cue-elicited craving engage in distorted thinking, overestimating the positive effects of smoking, which predisposes them to smoke.

Fortunately, even in these challenging circumstances, patients can do something to stop themselves smoking. Those who cope by changing what they are doing (for example, leaving the scene, eating something) or changing what and how they are thinking (for example, refocusing on why they want to quit or on a relaxing scene) are more likely to get through the testing situation without smoking. It is therefore vital that smokers who are planning to quit anticipate these challenges and prepare coping strategies to deal with them.

Although the probability of quitting successfully in any one attempt is low, many smokers do eventually become ex-smokers by making repeated attempts to quit. Figure 5.5 shows the cumulative probability of becoming an ex-smoker with increasing age in a large representative sample in England.

An unsuccessful attempt to quit does not doom a smoker to repeated failure. In fact, the number of previous quit attempts does not predict the chances of success of the next one.

Smokers who have tried and failed should try again, ideally after learning from their past failures by analyzing what went wrong. Smokers who have just failed in an attempt to quit may need a period of a few months or so to 'rest' and recover from that effort. After that, few of them give up on quitting; most are

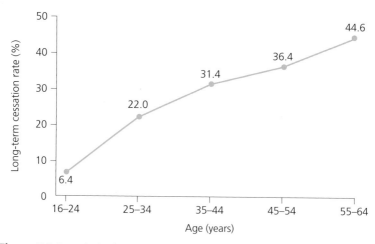

Figure 5.5 Cumulative long-term cessation rate (ex-smokers as a proportion of ever-smokers) in England as a function of age. Source: www.smokinginengland.info.

receptive to trying again, and most will do so within a few years. Most clinical trials of smoking cessation treatments (whether behavioral or pharmacological) are conducted on smokers with a history of repeated failures, so the treatments that demonstrate efficacy can help even battle-hardened smokers to quit.

Most smokers are unhappy about their smoking and want to stop; in the USA and the UK, about 40% report having tried to stop in the past year. Those who fail are highly likely still to be motivated to have another attempt, and some try to quit several times a year. Contrary to what is popularly believed, younger smokers are more motivated to stop and try to stop more often than older smokers. This may be because as smokers get older, it is the hard core who are least motivated to stop who remain as smokers. It could also be the case that experience of repeated failure at stopping over the decades reduces smokers' motivation to stop.

The process of smoking cessation

Surveys have found that approximately one-third of quit attempts involve trying to reduce cigarette consumption gradually. Perhaps surprisingly, these seem less likely to succeed than when smokers take the plunge and stop in one go. It would seem that the attempt fizzles out before the final quit date is reached. So once a smoker is ready to try to quit, it is best to advise him or her to cut out cigarettes in one go and then do everything possible to avoid lapsing.

For smokers who are not ready to quit in the immediate future, however, we now have good evidence that getting them to reduce the amount they smoke with the aid of either nicotine-replacement products or varenicline (see Chapter 7), with a view to quitting later, can be a very effective strategy.

It was thought for many years that smokers needed to go through a series of 'stages' before arriving at a quit attempt – they would think about stopping but not plan to stop in the near future, then they would plan to stop, then they would prepare to stop and finally they would make the attempt. Recent evidence indicates that this need not be the case. About half of all quit attempts are made without any pre-planning at all – the smoker does not even finish the pack of cigarettes he or she is smoking. What is more, these quit attempts are just as likely to succeed as ones that are planned in advance.

The process of smoking cessation can be usefully divided into two phases (Figure 5.6):

• the phase leading up to the quit attempt
• the phase after the quit attempt has started.

The phase leading up to the quit attempt is one in which a smoker struggles with the conflict between the knowledge of the harm that smoking does and continuing to smoke. A smoker experiences episodes of discomfort about his or her smoking when prompted to think about its harmful effects, excessive cost and feelings of stigma and so forth. The degree of discomfort when it occurs varies according to the nature of the beliefs and feelings and how salient they are at the time. Most of the time this discomfort is not sufficient to trigger a quit attempt because it is mitigated by the perception that quitting can be done at a later date, and it is countered by not wanting to give up the perceived benefits of smoking, together with anticipation of the difficulties and unpleasant consequences of trying to stop. Moreover, these discomforting thoughts and feelings are often overwhelmed by the moment-to-moment demands of everyday life, and by the draw of the next cigarette.

However, every now and then the discomfort will be stronger, the sense of urgency greater, the perceived benefits of smoking less important, and/or the anticipated difficulties less, swinging the balance of motivation in favor of making a quit attempt. If there is no reason to delay, the quit attempt will be put into effect immediately. Otherwise it will take the form of an intention to stop at some future time point, usually within a few days. Of course, the intention may change in the meantime, and intentions can vary from strong sustainable deliberate

Phase 1: While smoking

When the smoker is led to think about his or her smoking, he or she may feel a desire or need to stop that varies in strength and urgency arising from one or more of the following:

- Worry about health
- Dislike of financial cost of smoking
- Guilt or shame at smoking
- Disgust with smoking
- Hope for success at stopping
- Hope for improvement in health with stopping
- Hope for improved self-esteem with stopping
- Commitment to a remembered intention to make a quit attempt

These conflict with, and are mitigated by, a desire or need to smoke arising from one or more of the following:

- Anticipated enjoyment of a forthcoming cigarette
- Need for the forthcoming cigarette
- Concern about loss of self-esteem if the quit attempt fails
- Concern about unpleasant short-term effects of stopping
- Wanting or needing to hold on to the perceived benefits of smoking

Depending on the strengths of the competing desires and needs, the smoker may:

- Put the idea of stopping out of his or her mind
- Form an intention to stop at some vaguely conceived future time point
- Form a definite plan to stop at some future time point
- Decide to stop immediately

Phase 2: Once the quit attempt has started

On each occasion when the would-be ex-smoker is led to think about smoking, he or she experiences an urge to smoke arising from one or more of the following:

- A habit-driven impulse
- A need to smoke derived from 'nicotine hunger'
- A need to smoke derived from anticipated relief from negative mood
- A need to smoke derived from anticipated physical symptoms, e.g. mouth ulcers
- A desire to smoke derived from anticipated enjoyment or satisfaction
- A desire to smoke derived from anticipated benefits of smoking, e.g. weight loss

This competes with a desire or need for the smoker to stop himself or herself smoking that arises from one or more of:

- Commitment to the decision not to smoke
- Commitment to the identity of a non-smoker
- Worry about health
- Anticipated guilt or shame at having a cigarette
- Hope for improvement in health with stopping
- Anticipated disappointment at having wasted the effort expended thus far
- Anticipated effort required to acquire a cigarette

If the strength of the urge to smoke is greater than the inhibition arising from the desire or need not to smoke, and the opportunity to smoke is present, the would-be ex-smoker will:

- Smoke a cigarette but consider that the quit attempt is continuing
- Abandon the quit attempt but try to keep smoking within certain limits
- Abandon the quit attempt completely

Figure 5.6 The process of smoking cessation.

intentions to more fragile intentions that fail to survive even slight challenges. Research has found that the intention to quit does not follow a steady course building up to a cessation effort. On the contrary, such intentions seem to be quite volatile, changing from day to day. It is not known what triggers such abrupt changes, but the pattern suggests that clinicians should take advantage of any signs of interest in quitting, rather than waiting for such motivation to mature or postponing the attempt to some more opportune moment.

The phase after the quit attempt has started is one in which the smoker experiences urges to smoke arising from: habit; a need to smoke due to 'nicotine hunger'; a need to escape unpleasant feelings; missing the pleasures of smoking (including the loss of smoker identity/smoking with others); and feeling uncomfortable about physical effects of stopping, such as weight gain. These feelings and impulses are prompted by reminders and cues, and their strength depends on the nature of the underlying physiological and psychological processes as well as the context in which they occur. The motivation to smoke is countered by: the desire and need not to smoke that arises from the commitment to the quit attempt; anticipated shame and guilt from failure; anticipation of praise, respect and self-respect from success; a need to avoid adverse effects of smoking; and a desire to attain the health and financial benefits of stopping.

At any one moment, the balance between the forces motivating restraint and the motivations to smoke determines whether the would-be ex-smoker accepts the offer of a cigarette, goes out and buys a packet of cigarettes or engages in some other activity that leads to smoking. It is not just passive motivation that determines the outcome at such critical moments. When faced with a temptation to smoke, and if equipped with adequate motivation to avoid smoking, smokers can actively cope with the urge in order to avoid smoking. Coping, either by doing something or by changing the way one thinks in the moment – or, ideally, both – can prevent a lapse even in the face of a strong temptation.

If the would-be ex-smoker does smoke a cigarette in response to the immediate urge or need to smoke, usually he or she does not immediately abandon the quit attempt. It is regarded as an exception, and he or she plans to resume abstinence afterwards. Even after the quit attempt is abandoned, it can take weeks or even months before the previous pattern of smoking is re-established, and the smoker usually retains an interest in stopping at a future time point.

As time passes and the would-be ex-smoker succeeds in maintaining abstinence, the nicotine hunger abates, the withdrawal symptoms subside and the habit-driven urges become weaker. In many cases, the commitment to the plan of becoming a permanent ex-smoker strengthens because of the investment that has already gone into it, and the likelihood of

---

Key points – addiction to cigarettes

- Cigarette addiction involves powerful motivations to smoke that undermine and overwhelm the desire to avoid smoking because of its social, financial and health costs.
- Cigarette addiction stems primarily from nicotine dependence.
  - Repeated rapid intake of nicotine from cigarettes sets up a powerful association between smoking and situations in which smoking typically occurs.
  - It also creates 'nicotine hunger' so that when brain nicotine levels fall, the smoker experiences a need to smoke.
  - It creates unpleasant withdrawal symptoms, including mood disturbance, because of physiological adaptation.
- The withdrawal symptoms are relieved by smoking, thus generating the feeling of a need to smoke whenever these symptoms are experienced, even if they are caused by something else.
- Addiction to cigarettes is demonstrated by the fact that fewer than 5% of serious attempts to stop smoking succeed without behavioral support or pharmacological treatment.

relapse therefore decreases. However, anything that rekindles the motivation to smoke, whether it be a social situation, a stressful event or something more subtle, can lead to a lapse and then relapse if the counterbalancing motivation to exercise restraint is not activated and sufficiently strong.

Key references

Kozlowski LT, Porter CQ, Orleans CT et al. Predicting smoking cessation with self-reported measures of nicotine dependence: FTQ, FTND, and HSI. *Drug Alcohol Depend* 1994;34:211–16.

Tobacco Advisory Group. *Nicotine Addiction in Britain – a Report of the Tobacco Advisory Group.* London: Royal College of Physicians, 2000.

USDHHS. *The Health Consequences of Smoking – 50 Years of Progress. Nicotine Addiction. A Report of the Surgeon General.* Atlanta: United States Department of Health and Human Services, Centers for Disease Control and Prevention, National Center for Chronic Disease Control and Prevention, Office on Smoking and Health, 2014.

West R, Brown J. *Theory of Addiction*, 2nd edn. Oxford: Wiley-Blackwell, 2013.

Recording and using smoking as a vital sign

Smoking is linked to so many diseases that recording it is imperative in the diagnosis of a condition and in deciding its management. Failing to record smoking status and acting on the result is considered by leading professional organizations such as the UK's Royal College of Physicians and the American Medical Association to be tantamount to negligence. Smoking history is important in the diagnosis of chronic obstructive pulmonary disease (COPD). It can also be useful in the preliminary diagnosis of other smoking-related diseases and where a hidden psychiatric disorder is suspected.

Advising patients to stop

It is now recognized that all clinicians have a role to play in encouraging and aiding smoking cessation. This need not be time-consuming or confrontational if undertaken properly. Research has shown that brief opportunistic advice from a physician can trigger an attempt to stop smoking in about 40% of cases. If the smoker then attempts to quit with no treatment, he or she has only a 5% chance of long-term success. Hence, the overall effect of the physician's advice alone (without assistance) is to create one long-term ex-smoker for about every 50 people advised. This may seem like a very low figure, but when one considers that the advice can take as little as 30 seconds, that the cost, taking into account the physician's time, is no more than £10 or US$15, and that stopping smoking yields an average of up to 10 extra years of healthy life, then, bearing in mind that some smokers who stop will relapse and others who did not respond will stop later, the cost per healthy life-year gained can be as little as £1000 or US$1500. Taking into account the cost savings on smoking-related illness and time off work, brief advice to stop smoking actually results in a cost saving.

There are, of course, limits to what brief advice on its own can achieve. First of all, there may be a risk that repeatedly raising the subject of smoking with a patient may undermine the doctor–patient relationship, adversely affecting adherence to treatment regimens for other conditions and even causing a smoker to avoid seeing the doctor. Second, without effective treatment for nicotine dependence (see below), it is mostly less-dependent smokers who stop in response to brief advice from their physician. The more-dependent smokers are in greater need of stopping but are less likely to do so. Third, the law of diminishing returns appears to apply, so that smokers who have not responded to previous advice are less likely to respond the next time it is given.

For these reasons, national and international professional guidelines suggest that physicians aim to raise the issue of smoking with patients known to be smokers at least once a year. Figure 6.1 shows a flowchart of how such a consultation might progress. The goal is to trigger a quit attempt in as many smokers as possible and to encourage as many smokers as possible to use effective treatments to help that quit attempt succeed.

Encouraging quit attempts. The first task is to check whether the smoker has already given up (Figure 6.1). If not, then rather than berating the smoking or even advising the patient to stop, the evidence suggests that clinicians should just advise smokers that there are now effective methods to help with quitting and encourage the smoker to try one of these. If the smoker is not interested, the clinician simply closes the conversation by inviting the smoker to think about quitting and to get in touch if he or she changes his or her mind.

Note that this is very different from the traditional approach of advising smokers to stop and then talking about different methods of stopping if they show an interest. It seems that better results are obtained and the interaction with the patient is more positive if the clinician simply advises all patients about

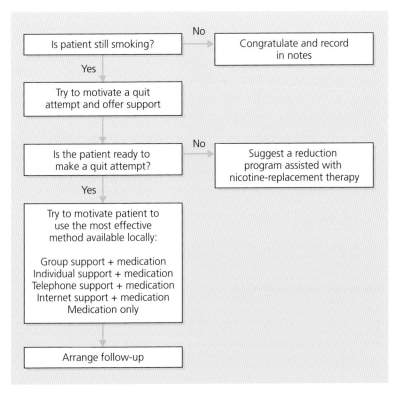

Figure 6.1 Providing brief advice to smokers to quit: a simple strategy for clinicians.

the best ways of stopping if they want to and encourage them to use one of them.

Enhancing success. If the smoker expresses an interest in stopping, attention switches to enhancing the efficacy of the quit attempt through treatment. The clinician should refer the smoker to a trained stop-smoking specialist (whether in-person services or those offered via telephone) if one is available, as he or she will be able to provide the full range of help. This may require nothing more than providing the smoker with a card or leaflet showing the telephone number. Smokers should also be encouraged to use pharmacological treatment (discussed below). If a trained specialist is not available but the physician is trained and can provide behavioral support, a schedule of appointments can be made to provide this help and support. If, however, the physician does not have the training or time to provide behavioral support, he or she should discuss appropriate medication and provide whatever help and support he or she can.

When discussing medication with the patient, the clinician needs to recognize that many smokers have already tried nicotine-replacement therapy (NRT) or varenicline (Champix/Chantix). Thus, he or she might say something like: 'The evidence is very clear that using medication doubles your chances of stopping for good. Even if you've tried it before, your chances of succeeding this time are still much better than if you try to stop cold-turkey'. There is evidence that NRT and varenicline are effective even for those who have previously been unsuccessful with it.

Training in smoking cessation and knowledge of the effects of smoking

As well as having a vital role in encouraging smokers to stop, referring them to cessation treatment services and prescribing medication to aid the quit attempt, clinicians must also be aware of the wide range of interactions between smoking and the clinical conditions that they manage. Smoking is not covered particularly well in undergraduate or postgraduate

Key points – the clinician and smoking

- Smoking is an essential vital sign; it is imperative that patients' smoking status be recorded and the record kept up to date.
- A physician's advice on smoking has a positive effect and need take as little as 30 seconds.
- The advice should focus, taking a small amount of time in routine consultations at least once a year, on telling all smokers about the best ways of stopping rather than berating smokers or just advising them to stop.

medical education. However, courses are available, and the situation is likely to improve over the next decade.

Several useful resources are available to assist in educating clinicians about smoking. Very useful websites containing resources in English include the UK National Centre for Smoking Cessation and Training's www.ncsct.co.uk, and the US National Cancer Institute's www.smokefree.gov. National guidelines are also available (see Key references).

Key references

AHRQ. *Treating Tobacco Use and Dependence, 2008 Update.* Rockville, MD: Agency for Healthcare Research and Quality, US Department of Health and Human Services, April 2013. www.ahrq.gov/professionals/ clinicians-providers/guidelines-recommendations/tobacco/clinicians/ update/index.html, last accessed 27 January 2016.

Fiore MC, Bailey W, Cohen S et al. *Treating Tobacco Use and Dependence.* Washington DC: United States Department of Health and Human Services (USDHHS), 2000.

NICE. *Smoking: tobacco harm-reduction approaches. NICE guidelines [PH45].* London: National Institute for Health and Care Excellence, June 2013. www.nice.org.uk/guidance/ph45, last accessed 29 February 2016.

NICE. *Smoking: supporting people to stop.* NICE Quality Standard (QS43). London: National Institute for Health and Care Excellence, August 2013. www. nice.org.uk/ guidance/qs43, last accessed 29 February 2016.

NICE. *Stop Smoking Services. NICE guidelines [PH10].* London: National Institute for Health and Care Excellence, February 2008. www.nice.org.uk/guidance/ph10, last accessed 29 February 2016.

RACGP. *Supporting Smoking Cessation. A guide for health professionals.* Melbourne: Royal Australian College of General Practitioners, 2011 (updated July 2014). www.racgp.org.au/your-practice/guidelines/smoking-cessation, last accessed 29 February 2016.

Tobacco Advisory Group. *Nicotine Addiction in Britain – a Report of the Tobacco Advisory Group.* London: Royal College of Physicians, 2000.

West R, McNeill A, Raw M. National smoking cessation guidelines for health professionals: an update. *Thorax* 2000;55:987–99.

Optimal treatment

Structured behavioral support combined with medication (nicotine-replacement therapy [NRT], bupropion [formerly amfebutamone] or varenicline) is the treatment of choice to aid smokers who want to quit. This combination can improve the chances of success of a quit attempt from 5% when unaided to more than 20% (Figure 7.1).

In the absence of an available program of structured behavioral support, medication plus limited behavioral support, such as might be feasible in routine consultations via a telephone quitline or through the internet, is an important treatment option.

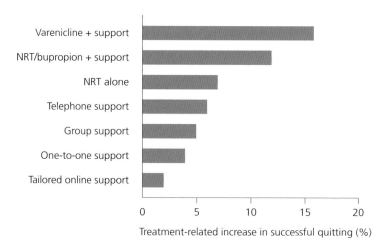

Treatment-related increase in successful quitting (%)

Figure 7.1 Estimated increase in percentage of quit attempts that succeed for at least 6 months with particular treatments, both medication and behavioral support (derived from Cochrane reviews of relevant randomized controlled trials). Note that dual-form NRT, involving use of a patch plus a faster-acting product (see later) can produce results comparable to varenicline. NRT, nicotine-replacement therapy.

Behavioral support

Research has consistently shown that a structured behavioral support program, whether conducted with groups of smokers, one-to-one (face-to-face) with a specialist or by telephone with a trained counselor, can significantly increase a smoker's chances of long-term success in stopping smoking. Many different face-to-face behavioral support programs are available, including some inpatient programs (though the incremental value of an inpatient program has not been demonstrated). Most follow a pattern of one or two pre-quit sessions, followed by regular sessions in the 4–6 weeks following the quit date.

Figure 7.2 shows a treatment plan in a typical smokers' clinic. The key elements are:
- sessions before the quit date
- a specified quit date
- a clear target of total abstinence
- medication as an integral part of the treatment plan unless contraindicated
- sessions at least weekly
- sessions for at least 4 weeks after the quit date
- discussion of a range of motivational devices to overcome urges to have a cigarette
- use of social motivation to enhance and maintain commitment
- education about situations that may provoke relapse
- presentation of a variety of means for coping with these situations
- recording of expired-air carbon monoxide to confirm abstinence at sessions after the quit date.

The following sections give a flavor of what the various sessions might involve.

Assessment session. Behavioral support programs typically begin with an assessment session in which the smoker's commitment to making a serious attempt to stop smoking is

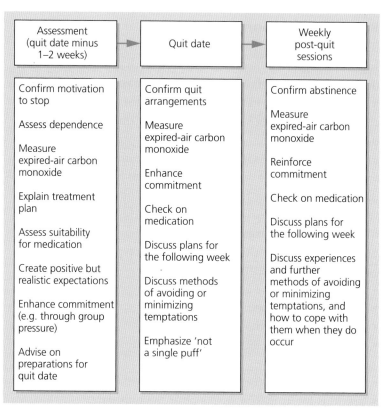

Figure 7.2 Treatment plan in a typical smokers' clinic.

confirmed, his or her level of dependence is gauged and the schedule of sessions is explained. Smokers may be asked to observe or monitor their smoking patterns in order to anticipate situations in which they may face temptations to smoke. At the assessment session a quit date, or date and time when the attempted abstinence will begin, is decided; this is usually 1–2 weeks in the future. Where medications (see below) are available and not contraindicated, they will usually form an integral element of the treatment package and the most appropriate form of medication will be determined during the assessment session. Several studies have demonstrated a benefit to initiating NRT for 1–2 weeks before the quit date, so NRT may be initiated at this stage. Bupropion and varenicline also need to be initiated before the quit date in order to build up to adequate blood levels.

Approaching the quit date. The choice of medication is reviewed if appropriate, and commitment to cessation is reinforced using a range of techniques. These might include making a verbal and/or written statement to the therapist or in front of the group. In a group setting, smokers may be paired up to provide each other with support during the following week. The counselor will emphasize the importance of not smoking at all (i.e. not having even a single puff on a cigarette) and will discuss ways of avoiding or minimizing temptations to smoke. The counselor will prepare smokers for the withdrawal symptoms they may experience, and discuss ways of coping with these.

After the quit date. Another session takes place a week or so after the quit date, and further sessions may be arranged weekly for a further 3–5 weeks. During these sessions the smoker's expired-air carbon monoxide concentration is measured. This serves two functions.

- It provides immediate verification that the smoker has remained abstinent at least on that day.
- It serves to boost the smoker's motivation by demonstrating improvement in a physiological marker.
  The smoker discusses his or her experiences with the counselor or support group, and any problems that are anticipated in the week ahead. Issues relating to the medication can also be discussed where appropriate.

Preventing relapse. Although behavioral support sessions typically run for 4–6 weeks after the quit date, further sessions are sometimes arranged at less frequent intervals in an attempt to prevent relapse. As yet, evidence has not shown that such sessions are helpful in preventing relapse. However, smokers like to know that the counselor will follow them up and retain an interest in their progress. The program of support can be given face-to-face or by scheduled telephone contacts.

Medication

Three forms of medication are typically available to assist smokers in attempts to quit and are licensed in at least some countries: bupropion, varenicline and NRT (Table 7.1).

TABLE 7.1

Medications to help smokers quit

Main contraindications	Comment
Bupropion (Zyban) – 150 or 300 mg/day	
History of, or predisposition to, seizures; pregnancy	Requires a prescription; may be slightly more effective than a nicotine patch but with risk of seizure of 1/1000
Varenicline (Champix, Chantix) – 0.5 or 1 mg/day after an initial period of dose escalation	
Pregnancy	Requires a prescription; studies have found superior efficacy to bupropion in unselected patients; reduces both urge to smoke and rewarding effect of a cigarette if a lapse occurs; main side effect is nausea; no evidence of increased risk of side effects in comparative studies, but spontaneous reports of neuropsychiatric side effects are higher than would be expected
Nicotine patch – 24 h or 16 h	
Caution on use in pregnancy and immediately following acute cardiac event*	Convenient and popular with smokers; available without prescription in some countries; some patches provide different doses for lighter and heavier smokers; most provide for a three-dose step-down program to taper nicotine dose over 10–12 weeks, though no evidence that this is required

(CONTINUED)

TABLE 7.1 (CONTINUED)

Nicotine gum – 2 mg or 4 mg

As above   Available without prescription; actual dose is much less than nominal dose; 4 mg gum recommended for smokers of 20/25 (UK/USA) or more cigarettes/day; smokers typically use too few pieces of gum and should be encouraged to use recommended amounts; for smoking cessation, gum may be used for relief of acute cravings

Nicotine inhalator – 1 mg/20 min use

As above   Prescription-only in the USA; supposed to replace habit of smoking; nicotine absorption is through the mouth, not the lungs, so is similar to that from nicotine gum

Nicotine sublingual tablet – 1 mg

As above   Similar absorption to 2 mg nicotine gum, but more discreet to use; not available in the USA

Nicotine lozenge – 1 mg, 2 mg or 4 mg

As above   Available without prescription; 2 mg tested in less-dependent smokers; 4 mg tested in more-dependent smokers; a 1 mg lozenge is also available; nicotine is delivered at similar speed to nicotine gum but a higher total dose is obtained

Nicotine nasal spray – 0.5 mg per spray

As above   Prescription-only in the USA; most rapid form of nicotine delivery among NRTs; highly irritant in nose at first; may be best used under supervision

*In many countries, most or all forms are described as contraindicated in pregnancy and in patients with heart disease, but guidelines recognize that the risk, if any, is much less than that from smoking, and suggest use under close supervision instead. Nicotine mouth spray and dissolvable strips are covered in the text.
NRT, nicotine-replacement therapy.

Bupropion and all forms of NRT have been shown to approximately double a smoker's chances of stopping successfully and remaining abstinent in the long term. Varenicline has greater efficacy overall than bupropion and is likely more effective than 'standard' use of NRT (see below for more details). These medications are of critical importance in the treatment of nicotine dependence.

Bupropion (brand name Zyban) is started 1 week before the quit date to allow steady-state levels to be reached in the blood. The usual dose is a single 150 mg tablet per day for the first week, increasing to two 150 mg tablets per day by the quit date. The medication is normally continued for a further 7–11 weeks, and there is evidence that it can prevent relapse for as long as 1 year if taken over such an extended period. However, it is not clear whether extending use long term improves the chances of abstinence beyond the period of drug administration.

The precise mode of action of bupropion is not known, but its effects are thought to arise from increased activity in dopamine and norepinephrine (noradrenaline) pathways in the central nervous system (CNS). Depletion of dopamine levels in the nucleus accumbens has been implicated in urges to smoke. Bupropion reduces the severity of withdrawal symptoms and the urge to smoke. Its potential as an aid to smoking cessation was discovered by chance when the drug (under the brand name Wellbutrin) was being used as an antidepressant. However, its effect on smoking cessation does not rely on its antidepressant actions and is not confined to smokers who are depressed.

There is evidence from one clinical trial that adding bupropion to varenicline (see below) increases smoking cessation rates in smokers of more than 20 cigarettes per day.

Varenicline (brand name Chantix in the USA, Champix elsewhere) was specifically designed to aid smoking cessation. It is modeled on the plant extract cytisine (discussed below) and is a partial agonist at the $\alpha_4\beta_2$ nicotinic acetylcholine (ACh) receptor believed to be involved in nicotine dependence. As a partial agonist, it increases activation in downstream neural pathways. This is sufficient to reduce the urge to smoke and the withdrawal symptoms but it does not reward or induce dependence itself. By binding to that receptor, varenicline prevents nicotine from attaching to it, thereby probably reducing the rewarding effect of smoking. In head-to-head trials, varenicline has been found to be more effective than bupropion. It has few contraindications, although close monitoring has been suggested when it is given to smokers with psychiatric conditions. It is more expensive than bupropion but, because it is more effective, the cost-effectiveness in terms of cost per life-year saved is similar to that for bupropion.

Following a spate of stories in the media, regulatory bodies in several countries have required the manufacturer to put warnings on the varenicline label about possible neuropsychiatric side effects. However, large-scale comparative studies and meta-analyses of randomized controlled trials involving many thousands of smokers have not shown an increased incidence of these effects. A meta-analysis has also reported an increased risk of cardiovascular events associated with varenicline use, but this did not take account of key confounding factors. Other meta-analyses have not shown a significant increase in such events.

Nicotine-replacement therapy is available in various forms, not all of which are available in all countries. All forms of NRT have been shown to reduce craving and withdrawal symptoms. Dosing typically begins on the quit date and continues for 8–12 weeks, depending on the product. Given that NRT simply replaces some of the nicotine that smokers had been getting from cigarettes, there are few genuine contraindications, and the products have been found to be safe for use by patients with a range of medical conditions, including heart disease.

Use in pregnancy is more controversial, because nicotine probably has some damaging effects on the fetus and randomized controlled trials have failed to show a benefit over placebo in terms of cessation – although one study did show an improvement in the health of the baby following birth. In general, the rational approach is to explain the risks to pregnant smokers and to suggest that they use NRT if the alternative would be to continue smoking. One study found that while just using one form of NRT did not improve quit rates during pregnancy, a combination of a transdermal patch and a faster-acting product such as chewing gum or inhalator (see below) was associated with higher quit rates.

Nicotine chewing gum was the first NRT to be developed and has been available in many countries for about 20 years. Two main doses are available, 2 mg and 4 mg, which typically yield about 1 mg and 1.5–2 mg nicotine, respectively. This is because not all the nicotine is released from the gum, and some of the released nicotine is swallowed and metabolized by the liver without ever reaching the general circulation. The 4 mg gum is recommended for people who smoke 20–25 cigarettes per day or more (the cut-off point depends on the country), or who smoke their first cigarette within 30 minutes of waking, while the 2 mg gum is directed at lighter and less-dependent smokers.

Smokers are advised to use 9–20 pieces of gum per day initially, tapering the frequency after 6 weeks. Although it is usually recommended that the gum is used at regular intervals rather than at the onset of craving (in response to a cue), it has been shown that the gum can help relieve acute craving when taken in response. In practice, many smokers use far too little gum to be of much benefit. This may be partly because the gum causes some irritation in the mouth and throat, and can produce nausea. It may also be because smokers are worried about absorbing too much nicotine. It is important to reassure smokers on both counts: the irritancy and nausea quickly resolve, and pure nicotine in these doses is not harmful. Another concern for many smokers is that they will become dependent on the gum. In practice, persistent use of the gum is uncommon, and dependence is quite rare, probably because the gum releases nicotine much more slowly than cigarettes. People who appear to have difficulty coming off the gum are typically those who were more dependent on cigarettes than other smokers and would almost certainly have gone back to smoking without the aid of the gum. In these cases, evidence shows that gum use tapers over a period of months or sometimes years. It is important to remember that the gum is relatively harmless, and even if users continue to chew it for many years, the health effects would be minimal, and certainly far smaller than the effects of smoking.

Nicotine lozenges are available in two formulations. One formulation from GlaxoSmithKline has been clinically proven and is available in 2 mg and 4 mg lozenges. Novartis market a 1 mg lozenge which is yet to undergo clinical trials. The nicotine is absorbed through the lining of the mouth, as it is from nicotine gum. The 2 mg and 4 mg lozenges deliver more nicotine than gum of the corresponding doses, because all the nicotine is released. The 4 mg lozenge has been tested only with more-dependent smokers (those who light up within 30 minutes of waking), while the 2 mg lozenge has been tested only with less-dependent smokers (those who first light up more than 30 minutes after waking). In both cases, the lozenges proved effective. The lozenges have also been shown to be effective in both light (≤ 15 cigarettes per day; 2 mg lozenge) and heavy (≥ 40 cigarettes per day; 4 mg lozenge) smokers.

Nicotine patches were the second form of NRT to be developed, prompted by the realization that many smokers were not using enough gum to obtain a therapeutic dose; the aim was therefore to provide nicotine in a more convenient and comfortable form. Several different patch technologies are available, but the essential principle is that nicotine is absorbed through the skin from a reservoir. Absorption is slow, and it takes 2–6 hours for blood nicotine levels to reach a plateau, depending on the brand of patch. In order to address morning nicotine cravings, some manufacturers have developed patches that are to be worn 24 hours a day. This means that blood nicotine levels are already high when the smoker wakes, and, in one comparative trial, a 24-hour patch demonstrated better control of craving than a 16-hour patch. However, comparative trials have not established whether wearing a patch for 24 hours is more successful in helping smokers to stop than wearing it for 16 hours and removing it at night. Some smokers experience sleep disturbance, sometimes associated with very vivid dreams, when wearing a patch overnight, and are best advised to remove the patch for sleep.

Nicotine nasal spray provides the most rapid form of nicotine delivery of any current NRT. A nicotine solution is sprayed as a metered dose of 0.5 mg into the nose. The user is advised to use one shot in each nostril, giving a total nicotine dose of 1 mg. The nicotine is absorbed through the permeable membrane of the nose, and a peak blood level is reached within 5–10 minutes. There is some evidence that the spray is most effective in more-dependent heavy smokers. Although smokers find the spray highly irritant at first, they become accustomed to it after a few days. There is no evidence of damage to the nasal membranes, even with long-term use.

Nicotine inhalators consist of a cartridge containing a nicotine-impregnated material. The cartridge is held in a plastic device like a cigarette holder. The user sucks air through the cartridge, where it draws off nicotine vapor. Despite the name of the device, nicotine is not really inhaled: the vapor condenses in the mouth and throat, whence it is absorbed into the bloodstream; it never reaches the upper airways or lungs. This means that the rate of nicotine delivery is similar to that with nicotine gum. The dose is variable, depending on the rate of puffing, but with one puff roughly every 10 seconds, 10 minutes' puffing can deliver about 1 mg nicotine. Thus, extremely frequent and persistent puffing is required to deliver an effective dose of nicotine. The delivery of nicotine also depends on temperature, dropping off below 10°C (50°F). The

rationale in support of the inhalator is that is goes further than other NRT products in replacing the behavioral and motor activity of smoking, although whether this confers an advantage in practice is not clear.

Nicotine sublingual tablets are small pellets that are held under the tongue while they dissolve. Each tablet delivers 1 mg nicotine and is similar in terms of absorption and overall dose to 2 mg nicotine gum. Clinical trials have shown the formulation to be effective as an aid to smoking cessation and in the relief of withdrawal symptoms and urge to smoke.

Nicotine mouth spray involves a container of nicotine solution that can be sprayed into the mouth – usually one dose into each cheek. It delivers 1 mg of nicotine per spray but much of this will not be absorbed.

Nicotine dissolvable oral strips are thin oral strips containing 2.5 mg of nicotine. They are placed on the tongue and dissolve within a few minutes. The amount of nicotine delivered into the bloodstream is much less than 2.5 mg, and the rate of nicotine absorption is not materially different from that seen for other oral forms.

Enhancing the effectiveness of nicotine-replacement therapy

The most important thing to know about NRT use is that a combination of nicotine patch plus one of the other faster-acting, products improves success rates and should be adopted as standard. In a large comparative trial, this combined approach was superior to bupropion (but was not tested against varenicline).

Studies also suggest that use of nicotine patches for 2 weeks before quitting improves the chances of success at stopping compared with the standard regimen of starting patch use on the quit day (even among patients who are not advised to reduce their smoking before quitting). There is also evidence that continued use of nicotine patches after a smoker has lapsed (i.e. has had limited episodes of smoking) can increase the chances of recovering abstinence.

Correct compliance with NRT regimens improves quit rates, so patients must be encouraged to use patches for long enough; users of oral forms need encouragement to use the products often enough to secure the full benefit.

It is clear that the benefit of NRT, as with any medication, depends on adequate dose and duration. Smokers who use NRT without the benefit of any instruction or counseling may be particularly likely to use too little for too short a time, undermining the medication's efficacy. It is imperative that smokers using NRT think of it as they would antibiotics – they must use the appropriate dose and for the appropriate duration to gain the benefit.

Who can benefit from pharmacological treatment?

Smokers and health workers sometimes believe that if a smoker has tried a medication once, without success, they have demonstrated themselves to be unresponsive, and should not try the same medication again. However, both varenicline and NRT have been shown to be effective even in those smokers who previously failed on the treatment, and the same may be true of bupropion. Varenicline and NRT have also been helpful to smokers who have not decided exactly when they will quit but are intending to quit at some point in the next few weeks. In addition, they have been found to be very effective in promoting cessation in patients who are not willing to quit in the next month but are willing to reduce their smoking with a view to quitting at some point in the next 3 months. Importantly, the efficacy of varenicline and NRT is not limited to highly dependent smokers; they have been demonstrated to help a wide range of daily smokers. Efficacy with non-daily smokers has not yet been demonstrated.

Smoking reduction

At any one time, a substantial proportion of smokers – about 50% in England – are trying to 'cut down' their cigarette consumption. Unfortunately, there is little evidence that this in itself results in a meaningful reduction in risk. Indeed, nicotine intake is similar for these smokers as for other smokers, even though the average cigarette consumption is slightly lower, probably because such smokers take in more from each cigarette by puffing more often and/or more deeply.

There is some evidence, however, that smokers who cut down are more likely to go on to quit. Several studies have also found that those who use NRT to help them cut down are more likely to quit subsequently than those given a placebo. This has led regulatory authorities in many countries, including the UK, to allow manufacturers to market some NRT products for the purpose of cutting down for months and then quitting. In this indication, NRT plays multiple roles: facilitating reduction of smoking, helping the smoker's transition to abstinence, and helping to sustain abstinence after the quit date.

The key message for clinicians is that if a smoker is not ready to quit but is willing to try to cut down with a view to quitting later, this should be encouraged and they should be advised to use varenicline or NRT to help them achieve this.

Electronic nicotine delivery devices

Electronic nicotine delivery devices (ENDS), of which the most common examples are electronic cigarettes (e-cigarettes), have increased rapidly in popularity in recent years. In England, where usage is tracked every month (www.smokinginengland. info) they are now the most popular aid to cessation and to smoking reduction.

E-cigarettes consist of a cartridge containing liquid (e-liquid) made up of water, propylene glycol or glycerine, and usually nicotine and flavorings, a battery, a heating element and some electronics. Many e-cigarettes are designed to look somewhat like cigarettes and they often have a tip with an LED that lights up when the user sucks on them. When the heating element is activated (usually by sucking on the end of the device), the e-liquid is vaporized and the vapor is drawn into the mouth. In this way, the devices can deliver nicotine and give much of the experience of smoking but without inhalation of the tar and poisonous gases arising from tobacco combustion. The vapor emerging from the user's mouth looks a little like tobacco smoke but is nearly odorless made up of low small amounts of the e-liquid constituents. As e-cigarettes do not burn tobacco, they do not produce the brew of toxic combustion products produced by conventional cigarettes.

There are a lot of myths about e-cigarettes and it is important for health professionals to know the facts.

- While it is not known whether they are completely safe, there is no doubt that they are orders of magnitude safer than smoking.
- While there are limited clinical trial data on their efficacy, the data available and a large population study strongly suggest that, on average, they have effectiveness similar to that of other nicotine products in aiding smoking cessation. Moreover, as they operate on the same principle as the various nicotine replacement products, there is every reason to expect they would be effective in supporting cessation. They may also aid cessation in smokers who have not succeeded with other methods.
- ENDS appear to be gaining greater popularity, which may allow them to make a substantial positive impact on population health.
- Contrary to what is implied by some public health advocates, current use of e-cigarettes by people, including adolescents, who have never smoked is rare and there is little evidence to suggest that they are acting as a gateway to smoking.
- Many e-cigarette brands are owned by tobacco companies and marketed in ways that are reminiscent of cigarette advertising.
- So called 'second-generation' e-cigarettes, which look less like cigarettes and use rechargeable batteries and refillable e-liquid tanks, offer greater possibilities for tailoring strength and flavors and work out cheaper. As with any battery charging, care should be taken not to charge them near flammable objects or oxygen in case of overheating.

Clinicians are frequently asked whether they would recommend e-cigarettes. In the light of the above, the best advice to smokers is to use a method of stopping that has a stronger evidence base, but if that does not appeal or is unsuccessful, then using an e-cigarette is a reasonable option.

E-cigarettes are very variable in the amount of nicotine they deliver and in the quality of manufacture. Potential users should therefore be advised to try different strengths and flavors to see if they can find one that seems to meet their needs. Major brands may have better control of manufacturing quality.

Other treatments

Many individuals and commercial organizations offer treatments for smoking, or gadgets that purport to help the smoker to break the habit. Reviews by the Cochrane collaboration are an excellent source of authoritative up-to-date information on the efficacy of techniques for smoking cessation (see Useful resources, pages 84–6).

- Hypnotherapy is popular but has not been found to have any specific effect beyond general advice and support.
- Acupuncture has also been studied but was not found to have any specific effect.
- Graduated filters are designed to filter out more and more of the smoke and nicotine over time, with smokers switching to increasingly powerful filters over a period of weeks. There has been little research into these, but the limited evidence available suggests that they do not improve a smoker's chances of stopping.
- St John's wort contains pharmacologically active compounds that might be expected to affect smoking. For example, it contains a chemical that inhibits the body's ability to break down nicotine. This means that a particular dose of nicotine produces higher levels in the blood when St John's wort is also present. This could enhance the effectiveness of NRT, or lead smokers to reduce the amount they smoke to avoid toxic effects. However, at present there are no published

trials showing a benefit in aiding permanent smoking cessation.

- Many commercial 'herbal' products and dietary supplements are claimed to assist in smoking cessation but we know of no case where the claims are supported by valid clinical research data (randomized controlled trials with appropriate outcome criteria).
- Antidepressants and other medications for psychiatric conditions have been tested for effects on smoking cessation. Nortriptyline, a tricyclic antidepressant, has been shown to aid cessation in well-controlled clinical trials; in fact it has a similar level of effectiveness to bupropion. It is cheap, and has been recommended for this use in New Zealand and the Netherlands.

Cytisine (Tabex) was the first medication to be licensed as an aid to smoking cessation and has been used in former Soviet-bloc countries since the 1960s. It is a plant extract that acts as a partial agonist at $\alpha_4\beta_2$ nicotinic ACh receptors, much like varenicline. There is now strong evidence from high-quality clinical trials that it is effective and safe. A great advantage is that, like nortriptyline, cytisine is extremely cheap. Unlike nortriptyline, it has no known serious side effects at the doses used, and so offers the prospect of a treatment that could be widely used in countries where the cost of other medications is prohibitive. In Poland it is sold over the counter and is the most commonly used smoking cessation medication.

Special patient groups

Pregnant smokers. Of all smokers, pregnant women have the greatest need to stop. As noted in Chapter 4, the risks are not only to the life of the fetus or infant: the damage carries on into adulthood. Stopping smoking at any stage in pregnancy improves the health of the fetus compared with continuing to smoke.

There is good evidence that structured behavioral support programs delivered by trained specialists can improve pregnant smokers' chances of stopping for the duration of the pregnancy. In contrast, less intensive support delivered by midwives or other healthcare staff has not been found to be effective.

The major problem appears to be that many pregnant smokers are reluctant to admit to health professionals that they smoke, and only a small proportion are willing to receive behavioral support. Ideally, clinicians should ask about smoking in a way that enables women to admit to it without fear of stigmatization, and behavioral support services should be made as accessible as possible. One approach is to ask whether the mother-to-be has recently stopped smoking, and to recommend behavioral support to new 'ex-smokers' as well as current smokers. Given the health gains if a pregnant smoker manages to stop, it would even be cost-effective to deliver behavioral support in the woman's own home. Importantly, even among women who stop during pregnancy, there is a very high risk of relapse after birth; accordingly, such women should be provided with behavioral support and, if necessary, pharmacological treatment to avoid relapse.

As noted earlier, NRT has not been found in clinical trials to improve cessation rates but there is evidence from a large non-randomized comparative study that dual form NRT (transdermal patch plus one of the other products) may improve success rates.

Hospital inpatients. There are many reasons for treating hospital inpatients as a special case among smokers. For those undergoing surgery, smoking cessation provides short-term benefits in terms of postoperative recovery and wound healing. In addition, hospitals should be smoke free; a policy that benefits all patients and staff, smokers and non-smokers. Many of the patients will be suffering from smoking-related diseases, so the risks of continuing to smoke can be made personally relevant. Clinical trials have found that behavioral support for inpatients can improve smoking cessation rates if the support is sustained beyond the hospital stay.

Psychiatric patients. Prevalence of smoking is higher in psychiatric patients than in the general population, and the level of dependence is greater among those who do smoke. Psychiatric patients are just as motivated to stop smoking as other smokers and it is good clinical practice to offer support for stopping on a regular basis to all smokers, which they can take up if they wish to. There is some evidence that varenicline can help patients with severe psychiatric illness to stop, at least for several months. Otherwise it makes sense to offer dual form NRT and also to encourage psychiatric patients who cannot stop to reduce their smoking with the aid of NRT.

Individuals with alcohol use disorder are very likely to smoke, and to smoke heavily. Smokers with comorbid alcohol or drug problems have lower success rates in quitting. There has been some concern among clinicians that trying to quit smoking while also trying to stop drinking could endanger efforts at sobriety. However, several studies have shown that quitting smoking does not hinder success in alcohol treatment and may in fact enhance it.

Young smokers. The younger a smoker is when he or she stops, the greater the chance of a full recovery of life expectancy. Adolescent smokers quickly develop dependence, so behavioral support and medication would seem to be appropriate in some cases. Unfortunately, there is no clear evidence for the effectiveness of these treatments in adolescents. One problem may be instability in young smokers' determination to stop, even when they initiate a quit attempt. This is currently an active area of research.

Key points – treatments to aid smoking cessation

- A structured behavioral support program involving several sessions concentrated in the first few weeks after the quit date can significantly increase smokers' chances of stopping permanently.
- Sustained-release bupropion hydrochloride (Zyban) and nicotine-replacement therapy (NRT, in the form of chewing gum, transdermal patches, nasal spray, inhalator, lozenges, sublingual tablets, mouth spray or dissolvable oral strips) increase smokers' chances of stopping considerably.
- The highest quit rates can be achieved with either varenicline (Chantix/Champix) or dual-form NRT (patch plus one of the other forms of NRT).
- NRT, varenicline and bupropion are among the safest medicines available, although bupropion carries a small risk of seizure and allergic reaction (about 1/1000).
- Electronic cigarettes have become very popular and may help many smokers to stop smoking. They are much safer than conventional cigarettes, even if used long term. Concerns exist around the way some of them are being marketed and the variability in quality.
- Nortriptyline and cytisine are both effective at helping smokers to stop and are very cheap. Cytisine (available in much of Central and Eastern Europe for several decades and available over the counter) offers a safe and effective low-cost treatment that can be given with minimal supervision. It has yet to receive a marketing license in most of the world.
- A combination of behavioral support and medication quadruples the chances of a successful quit attempt; these treatments are among the most cost-effective life-preserving interventions available to health professionals.
- Hypnotherapy and acupuncture have received little research attention in relation to smoking cessation; to date, no specific effect in aiding smoking cessation has been found.

Key references

Fiore MC, Bailey W, Cohen S et al. *Treating Tobacco Use and Dependence*. Washington: United States Department of Health and Human Services (USDHHS), 2000.

NICE. *Smoking: acute, maternity and mental health services. NICE guidelines [PH48]*. London: National Institute for Health and Care Excellence, November 2013. www.nice.org.uk/guidance/ph48, last accessed 29 February 2016.

NICE. *Smoking cessation in secondary care overview. NICE Pathway*. www.pathways.nice.org.uk/pathways/smoking-cessation-in-secondary-care, last accessed 29 February 2016.

Tobacco Advisory Group. *Nicotine Addiction in Britain – a Report of the Tobacco Advisory Group*. London: Royal College of Physicians, 2000.

Tobacco smoking is a highly toxic form of nicotine use. Although nicotine itself appears to carry minimal risk of serious disease, tobacco smoking is deadly, contributing to dozens of diseases that cause disability and death. Without effective intervention, cigarette smoking is expected to have killed some 520 million people worldwide by 2050.

Fortunately, many governments around the world are beginning to wake up to the magnitude of the problem, and are developing tobacco control programs. Most, although not the USA, have signed the Framework Convention on Tobacco Control – an international treaty setting out national obligations to reduce the harm caused by tobacco. Table 8.1 lists the main national obligations included in the treaty.

Unfortunately, the health services in most countries have not been geared up to provide evidence-based support for quitting, even very low-cost clinical programs that could be incorporated into existing clinical services.

In countries that do have comprehensive smoking cessation programs, the challenge is in ensuring that smokers make full use of these services. Preventing young people from taking up smoking is also vital, although an impact on death rates will not become apparent for several decades. While research on improving treatments for smoking-related disorders continues, smoking cessation remains our best hope for reducing the burden of tobacco-related death and disease over the next 50 years.

If higher rates of smoking cessation are to be achieved, concerted action is required on all fronts: fiscal, legislative, educational and clinical. The challenge for physicians is to:
- develop clinical interventions that improve on the success rates of existing methods
- encourage more attempts to stop smoking

TABLE 8.1

National obligations under the Framework Convention on Tobacco Control

Signatories will:

- ban the promotion of tobacco products
- require large health warnings on all tobacco product packaging
- ban deceptive labeling such as 'low tar'
- ban smoking in indoor public areas and workplaces
- implement specific measures to combat tobacco smuggling
- consider using taxation as a means of reducing tobacco consumption
- establish a body to regulate tobacco products
- require disclosure of tobacco product ingredients
- consider litigation to make tobacco companies pay for the harm caused by their products
- endeavor to include tobacco cessation treatment in national health programs
- seek to prohibit distribution of free tobacco products
- prohibit sales of tobacco products to minors

Reproduced with permission of Oxford University Press from West R. Tobacco control: present and future. *Br Med Bull* 2006;77–8:123–36.
See also World Health Organization. Framework Convention on Tobacco Control. Geneva: WHO, 2003.
www.who.int/tobacco/framework/WHO_FCTC_english.pdf

- make greater use of effective treatments so that the proportion of attempts that are successful increases considerably.

This chapter briefly discusses some of the more promising lines of inquiry.

Improved forms of nicotine-replacement therapy

It seems reasonable to suppose that if a pure nicotine delivery system could be found that was almost as efficient as the cigarette and also as palatable, it would be more effective than the current generation of nicotine-replacement therapy (NRT) products in helping smokers to quit. However, it also seems likely that smokers would transfer their dependence to this product. Nevertheless, even if smokers continued to use such a product indefinitely, there would be minimal health risks, so this is an important area for development.

Ensuring effective use of nicotine-replacement therapy

There is now evidence that in countries where it has been studied, such as the UK, use of NRT bought over the counter and used without any professional support is not improving smokers' success rates. There is an urgent need to find out why and to take steps to ensure that smokers gain the benefit they expect. It is possible that these smokers are not using enough of the product or not using it for long enough for it to be effective. In that case, cheap scalable interventions to improve adherence to medication instructions could make a substantial difference.

New drugs to aid cessation

The commercial success of varenicline, NRT and bupropion has prompted many pharmaceutical companies to examine other medications that may help smokers to quit. The cannabinoid antagonist rimonabant showed some efficacy in aiding smoking cessation, its main feature being that it appeared to reduce post-cessation weight gain. Unfortunately, the clinical trials showed some evidence of cardiac toxicity and the drug has not been brought to market. However, the principle of action has been established and may spawn other drugs.

Work is also under way on a number of nicotine 'vaccines' that aim to prevent nicotine being taken up into the CNS, in order to dampen its effects there and thus make quitting or staying abstinent easier. To date, no vaccine has been found to be effective in clinical trials but the principle is intriguing and research continues.

Increasing use of traditional treatment services

A smoker's chances of stopping successfully without help are less than 5% in any given quit attempt. If that smoker attends a smokers' clinic and receives behavioral support and medication, the chance rises to 20%. However, at present only about 3% of smokers take advantage of these clinics in the UK each year, even though they are provided free of charge. Similarly, use of telephone counseling services in the USA is very low. Raising it to 10% would have an important effect on public health. The challenge is to find ways to increase uptake. Some studies have shown increased uptake when the clinician directly connects the patient to treatment services (e.g. arranging for a quitline counselor to call).

Novel channels for delivery of treatment services

So far, smoking cessation services have been delivered via traditional clinical channels, often modeled on mental health services, such as one-to-one meetings with a counselor, or group meetings with other smokers. Many smokers find these forms of treatment unappealing, and their availability is often limited. Studies are beginning to demonstrate the efficacy of treatment delivered through other channels, for example by means of telephone helplines, computer-tailored materials, the internet and smartphone apps.

Telephone helplines have proven to be effective, when provided by a trained counselor following evidence-based protocols. Telephone counseling that depends on smokers' initiative to call for help ('hotlines') is under-used and not as effective as counseling programs that schedule regular calls, paralleling the structure of face-to-face counseling.

A systematic review of randomized controlled trials has concluded that internet-based interventions can aid cessation but many do not and it is not clear what features make an effective internet support program. A very large randomized trial in the UK found that an open-source internet intervention called StopAdvisor increased quit rates in blue-collar smokers

(smokers in manual jobs) but not white-collar smokers (professionals). It had been specifically developed to appeal to the former group.

Although more than 200 stop-smoking apps are available, very few have data on their effectiveness. Most of them are unlikely to be effective given that they do not use evidence-based behavior change techniques. However, this is an active area of research and the situation is likely to change.

Key points – future trends

- If the pandemic of death from lung disease and cardiovascular disease is to be controlled, millions of smokers must quit.
- Price increases and mass media campaigns play a crucial role in motivating attempts to stop smoking.
- Effective treatments are available to support quit attempts; a major challenge lies in finding ways to get these treatments to the majority of smokers.
- In many countries, affordable and scalable systems need to be developed to ensure that smokers are offered evidence-based support for stopping as a matter of routine.
- In countries that have comprehensive smoking cessation programs, such as the UK and the USA, the main challenge is to ensure that smokers make full use of such services.
- More effective treatments, and treatments to help smokers who are not currently being helped, are focuses for current and future research.

Useful resources

UK

Action on Smoking and Health
Tel: +44 (0)207 404 0242
enquiries@ash.org.uk
www.ash.org.uk

Association of Respiratory Nurse
Specialists
Tel: +44 (0)7740 117902
info@arns.co.uk
www.arns.co.uk

British Lung Foundation
Helpline: 03000 030 555
www.blf.org.uk/support-for-you/
smoking/why-should-i-quit

British Thoracic Society
Tel: +44 (0)20 7831 8778
bts@brit-thoracic.org.uk
www.brit-thoracic.org.uk

Cancer Research UK
Tel: 0300 123 1022
www.cancerresearchuk.org

National Centre for Smoking
Cessation and Training
Tel: +44 (0)20 3137 9071
enquiries@ncsct.co.uk
www.ncsct.co.uk

National Institute for Health
and Care Excellence
Tel: 0300 323 0140
nice@nice.org.uk
www.nice.org.uk/guidance/
lifestyle-and-wellbeing/smoking-
and-tobacco

NHS Smokefree
www.nhs.uk/smokefree

Smoking in England
www.smokinginengland.info

Society for the Study of
Addiction
Tel: +44 (0)113 855 9559
www.addiction-ssa.org

USA

Action on Smoking and Health
Tel: +1 202 659 4310
info@ash.org
www.ash.org

American Association for
Respiratory Care
Tel: +1 972 243 2272
info@aarc.org
www.aarc.org
www.aarc.org/resources/clinical-
resources/tobacco-resources

American Cancer Society
Tel: 1 800 227 2345
www.cancer.org

American Lung Association
Tel: 1 800 548 8252
info@lung.org
www.lung.org
www.ffsonline.org

American Society of Addiction Medicine
Tel: +1 301 656 3920
email@asam.org
www.asam.org

American Thoracic Society
Tel: +1 212 315 8600
atsinfo@thoracic.org
www.thoracic.org
www.thoracic.org/advocacy/tobacco-control

Centers for Disease Control and Prevention
Tel: 1 800 232 4636
www.cdc.gov/tobacco

COPD Foundation
Tel (info): 1 866 316 2673
info@copdfoundation.org
www.copdfoundation.org

National Cancer Institute
Tel: 1 800 422 6237
www.cancer.gov/about-cancer/causes-prevention/risk/tobacco/smoking-cessation-hp-pdq

Smokefree.gov
Quit line: 1 877 448 7848
www.smokefree.gov

Society for Research on Nicotine and Tobacco
Tel: +1 608 443 2462
www.srnt.org

United States Surgeon General
Tel: +1 202 205 0143
ashmedia@hhs.gov
www.surgeongeneral.gov/priorities/tobacco

University of Wisconsin Center for Tobacco Research and Intervention
Quit line: 1 800 784 8669
www.ctri.wisc.edu/smokers

International
Australian Association of Smoking Cessation Professionals
Tel: +61 (0)2 9351 0816
admin@aascp.org.au
www.aascp.org.au

Chronic Obstructive Pulmonary
Disease Association (Singapore)
info@copdas.com
www.copdas.com

International Primary Care
Respiratory Group
Tel: +44 (0)1224 743753
execofficer@the ipcrg.org
www.theipcrg.org

The Lung Association (Canada)
Toll-free: 1 888 566 5864
Tel: +1 613 569 6411
www.lung.ca

Lung Foundation Australia
Toll-free: 1 800 654 301
Tel: +61 (0)7 3251 3600
enquiries@lungfoundation.com.au
www.lungfoundation.com.au

QuitNet
https://quitnet.meyouhealth.com

Quit Now (Australia)
Quitline: 13 7848
quitnow@health.gov.au
www.quitnow.gov.au

South African Thoracic Society
Tel: +27 (0)21 650 3050
sarj@iafrica.com
www.pulmonology.co.za

Treatobacco.net
www.treatobacco.net

WHO Tobacco Free Initiative
Tel: +41 (0)22 791 21 11
www.who.int/tobacco/en

FastTest

You've read the book ... now test yourself with key questions from the authors

- Go to the FastTest for this title
  FREE at fastfacts.com

- Approximate time **10 minutes**

- For best retention of the key issues, try taking the FastTest before and after reading

Biographies and disclosures

Robert West has been researching tobacco use since 1982 and is coauthor of the English National Smoking Cessation Guidelines and a popular book for smokers called The SmokeFree Formula (www.smokefreeformula.com). His current research includes clinical trials of new smoking cessation treatments, studies of the acute effects of cigarette withdrawal and population studies of smoking patterns (see www.rjwest.co.uk).

Professor West undertakes paid research and consultancy for and receives hospitality and travel funds from manufacturers of smoking cessation medicines.

Saul Shiffman is a psychologist who has studied tobacco use since 1973. His research focuses on nicotine dependence and its development, the nicotine withdrawal syndrome, and behavioral and pharmacological treatments for smoking, with a particular emphasis on smoking relapse and relapse prevention. Professor Shiffman is a Fellow of the American Psychological Association (in Health Psychology, Psychopharmacology and Addictions), the American Psychological Society and the Society for Behavioral Medicine.

Professor Shiffman consults to Niconovum (which markets smoking cessation products), and to Reynolds vapor (e-cigarettes), both subsidiaries of RJ Reynolds Tobacco, and has an interest in a company developing new smoking cessation medications.

Index

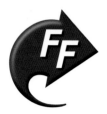

Fast Facts – the ultimate medical handbook series covers over 60 topics, including:

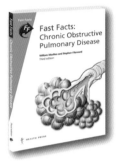

Fast Facts:
Chronic Obstructive
Pulmonary Disease

William MacNee and Stephen I Rennard
Third edition

Fast Facts:
Acute Coronary
Syndromes

Paul A Gurbel, Udaya S Tantry, Kurt Huber

Fast Facts:
Obesity

David Haslam and Gary Wittert
Second edition

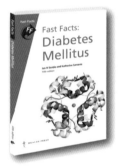

Fast Facts:
Diabetes
Mellitus

Ian N Scobie and Katherine Samaras
Fifth edition

Fast Facts:
Hypertension

Fast Facts:
Depression

Mark Haddad & Jane Gunn
Third edition

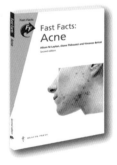

Fast Facts:
Acne

Alison M Layton, Diane Thiboutot and Vincenzo Bettoli
Second edition

Fast Facts:
Asthma

Stephen T Holgate and Jo A Douglass
Fourth edition

Fast Facts:
Liver
Disorders

Thomas Mahl and John O'Grady
Second edition

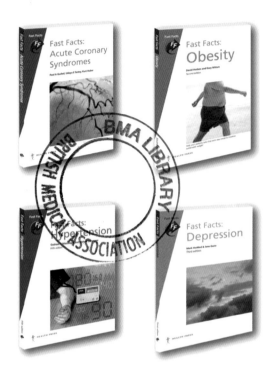
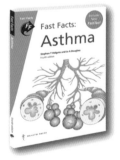
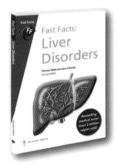

fastfacts.com